Don't Wish For It, Work For It!

Edited by Gareth Price & Liz Price

Contents

Foreword: David Evans

If you visit the self-help section in any good bookshop you will find countless books on exercise, nutrition, cooking, diets, lifestyles and much, much more. All these books have one thing in common, they are fundamentally about 'change' - making an improvement to your lifestyle, to your future, to your health, well-being or all-round life quality.

The challenge with many of them is that they are designed, in one way or another, to persuade you to subscribe to something, to buy into their cause and, in some cases, their product. This book is different - we want you to 'buy' into something completely different.

First though, let's talk about a word that is special, a word that sells thousands of products, stories, ideals, films, movies, make-believe the world over, a word that encapsulates all areas of human imagination - 'inspiration'.

What is inspiration? Inspiration is an almost physical response, caused by our very human elements, our mind, our brain, our breathing and is displayed by a single physical response, a sharp sudden intake of air. Have you ever felt surprised so much you become startled? Have you ever become so overwhelmed by a story that it gives you goose bumps?

True inspiration takes place at the heart of human endeavour, in the feats of local people, fired up by a cause, a mission, a challenge. Many years ago, I had the privilege of helping the local Bolton Hospice and an incredible woman called Leigh. She was an inspirational CEO determined to bring change to an organisation that every day is asked to deliver some of the best care available to its patients. People of all walks of life step up and volunteer and bring the best of themselves for those who cannot. The hospice, in Bolton, is full of stories of local people, like you and I, taking on challenges, asking what is possible, sometimes for ourselves, most often for others.

That difference that I mentioned earlier, is local inspiration, people who give their time and commitment to challenges to prove things to themselves, to do things that inspire others, to do things that, by their very nature, encourage others to do the same, however big, or small, the challenge.

Meeting the author

I first met Gareth at David Lloyd Leisure in Bolton many years ago, he was working for a huge construction company and was obsessed by challenges and raising funds for local causes. The challenge at the time was Kilimanjaro. He was a stubborn man, persistent, and determined to ensure that no stone was left uncovered in the pursuit of exploring his physical potential.

A Coffee Shop Dream: 'Build it and they will come'

Gareth and I got to know each other, he was intrigued by my profession and wanted to know about the things that RLC Coached around the world. We spoke about **M**indset, **E**xercise, **N**utrition and yo**U**, something that we have had many conversations about. The one thing that we always agreed on was that the first step is the one that counts.

During one conversation, Gareth shared that he was going to leave his job due to circumstances that were changing his life. In this process, he wanted to take control of his situation and the changes he was experiencing. He talked about opening a spinning studio like no other, he already knew the details - no mirrors,

4

no weights area, no machines, so people could feel safe in the environment; a place for community, a place to start.

There was one comment I made to Gareth that day that, he reminded me several months later, was particularly telling - "if you are obsessed about something and commit to it fully, more than anything else in your life, if you build it they will come". The phrase is from the film, Field of Dreams, where a man builds a baseball stadium in the middle of corn fields and the metaphoric voice keeps saying this phrase to the man who is obsessed and, of course, people came.

Several months later, Gareth and I met again, where he announced that he had done it. He had opened an alternative exercise studio in Bolton Town Centre and people were indeed coming. From that one act, that one moment of time, Gareth started something, he started a journey where some of the stories in this book are situated. One act, one moment, one level of commitment, one complete all-in decision that allowed him to not only do something he was determined to do, It also, unknown to him at the time, inspired many others to do the same. To take that first step towards something - a goal, a challenge, a run, a ride, a walk, a charity event and much more.

The stories here are of people like you and me who are not elite athletes, we are not the best of the best (though some are very good indeed), we are just people who are determined to answer the challenge in a way that forces us to find out what it is we are capable of. All the people at V1ntage studio, who have stood up and taken on a challenge, all have answered 'YES' first, then asked what is the question?

Gareth who has done three full Ironman UK, Bolton events, countless walking challenges, many, many, huge cycle rides which all started with his first step. Even with a replaced knee, he has battled pain, been stubborn, determined and persistent and has inspired many people into action - action that they say has allowed them to embrace more of their lives and themselves.

As you read this book we ask that you embrace the stories, enjoy the rollercoaster and challenges that people have put themselves through, learn about how they faced difficulty and overcame it.

As a Coach, Author and Keynote Speaker it would be remiss of me not to ask three simple questions of you the reader. These questions are about application, about thinking through your experience of the stories that you read.

Question **1** - What **action** could you take today?

Question **2** - What **one thing** could you change today that would enable a better future?

Question **3** - What could you do to inspire someone close to you to take the first step?

Introduction

Dave is right, there is a vast array of self-help books available these days, in book stores, online, in eBook format, on social media and in blogs. There's almost certainly motivational material in places I don't even know about, both virtual and in the real world and I'm really pleased that you've decided to read our book. You might be wondering, though, what makes this book different and why *is* there so much motivational material out there?

Well, for ten years I've wanted to write *this* book and for ten years before that I've wanted to write *a* book, but never really known what it was going to be about. I've always enjoyed writing when I've had the time. So, why has it taken me this long?

It's ironic, but it took my sister telling me to 'practice what I preach' and take a first step - to simply give it a go, and, with her help, that is exactly what I've done.

Our conversation on that day was ironic because it is the same conversation I have with people almost every day of my life, and this was all it took to persuade me to get started. My sister made it sound easy and, given that she has some experience of publishing, it helped to know she was onside with the project.

And here's why I use this example as a metaphor for why and how this book came about - its very reason for existence. **Everyone, needs a bit of help to do something that they think is beyond them**.

This helps explain why there's so much motivational material out there. I do wonder, though, how many authors of motivational books like this one, truly practice what they preach.

I can promise you that finally, after 61 years I only preach that which I practice!

It is my hope, that this book will help you to achieve whatever it is that you aspire to do. I would like to help you go beyond the 'dream' phase and turn whatever it is into a reality. Because, and sure it's a cliché, unless you have a go, the project is an inevitable failure!

Too late in my life, and that truly is my only regret these days, I've started to have a go at things that I am excited by and that scare me. I wish I'd been bolder when I was younger. Why didn't I you may ask, well it doesn't matter now because I'm not interested in the past really, especially where negatives are concerned.

What you'll not find here, however, are thousands of words about planning and scheming techniques. Rather, here, you'll find some brilliant examples of real people and their real stories, to show you that ordinary folk like you and me can achieve amazing things, simply by putting one foot in front of the other and having a go - having a go and staying focused on the end goal, rather than being scared off by the fear of failure

For the sake of scene setting, let's assume it's New Year. As it goes, I'm writing this chapter at New Year 2017/8, so that's easy for me to say. Right now, everyone is full of best intent, full of exciting ideas. Planning and plotting how to make their year a big success. Let's jump forward a few months, I know, you may scoff at this classic Neuro Linguistic Programming behaviour, but stay with me.

How many years have you got to March 1st and relinquished those best intentions, worse still, forgotten what they even were! I know, I'm with you, me too. Many times. Shit happens, that's how it is. Things change in everyone's lives, that's for sure. Those changes can disrupt your best intentions. So, without inviting you to recount your favourite story of success or failure, let's just agree this one thing

If you want something enough, you'll start the journey. The tough bit, is sticking to it. Whatever it is - the hard part is seeing it through.

There are lots of great stories in this book and some of them are mine. Some of the stories I'll relate are about my own experiences, these stories might, though, run the risk of having you shout out that I'm super athlete that's wired differently to you (I do enjoy the occasional extreme physical challenge as you will find out), but please be assured I am not elite in any way! I am just an average dude, trying to enjoy my life and wanting to share my thoughts on how to succeed. I want to normalise some of the epic challenges I've done and persuade you that anything really is possible.

First, though, I must tell you - and I'm shouting loud in your ear right now - that you need to believe in yourself, you need to understand what you're capable of. To do that, maybe ask yourself what aspect of your goal is actually totally impossible. Then think again, is it really impossible or just a challenge. If your goal is SMART, then you can do it.

Specific, **M**easurable, **A**chievable, **R**ealistic and **T**ime framed.

I've found it so exciting when I've thought about elements of my challenges in detail and realised it's just about doing things in small steps. Break it down. Like a jigsaw. After all, what's the difference between a child's 25-piece jigsaw and a 2000-piece brain twister, the answer is nothing, but patience and time.

Put to one side technique and skill and the worst case scenario will be learn as you go. I love this quote that I've heard Dave Evans use on more than occasion 'Build the parachute on the way down'

Here's where you've got to trust me. It really is that simple. It is, I would very strongly suggest, simply about tenacity and determination. In addition, you will inevitably need time and commitment and energy to fuel your body. You need your head set right. You need a **MENU** for success. You need your **M**IND, right, you need to embrace **EXERCISE** and you need to work on your **NUTRITION**, and then you'll begin to discover the best version of yo**U**. A formula for success - A MENU.

Still, I'm keeping it simple. And that's because it is. Here's another very popular cliché for you.

Impossible, is nothing. It's a cliché yes but when I really believe in!

What are the things you need to help you stay focused on your goal? What will prevent you from quitting? Whatever your goal is, you will have times when you want to do something better, something more fun, something less demanding.

Sometimes, it's easy to tell yourself it's ok to step down. That moment when you say, 'I'm not doing what I need to do today, I'm not doing what I said I would do!' And you might say that because you've got something that might seem more pleasurable at a given moment in time.

I'm here to tell you the pleasure is often short lived and the guilt of the 'quit action' is long lasting and damaging to your mindset. So, why not just do what you said you'd do and delete the debate in your head. Find a way to delete the debate as you hear yourself saying 'you know what, I'm not fancying this today' stop the inner voice from destroying the progress. The inner voice cares not a jot for your goals. It strikes when you are vulnerable!

Delete the debate.

Who can defeat the wicked inner voice? You're maybe saying to yourself right now, yeah, that's the problem. Who can? How can I keep it quiet, what's the secret to success? It's simple, you are the secret to your own success. You've just got to follow the plan. Keep following the route you plotted. Your **SMART** goals don't allow for the Inner voice to succeed when it's making negative noise.

Delete the debate. Take the T out of can't and **focus on CAN**. Your grasp of total positivity is a huge variable. Different days you'll be better at it than others. Some days you'll not even think of making positivity your mantra. That's ok. Same here!

It's ok to stumble. It's not ok to stay down and it's not ok to look back and think you've failed. It's essential that you erase the negativity and start again. No matter how you despair at whatever you've missed doing. Turn your head forwards and look to what you can do now and today.

Where's the magic here?

A simple answer – there is none. There are no magic formulas in my opinion. I'm just one man. I have a view. I am surrounded in my life by some very positive people. Sure, there are, and there will in the future, people who only seem to hoover my positivity, those that seem to enjoy being in a world of negativity where it becomes easy to bail, quit and let things slide, but I want you to think about this positivity rule.

The more positive you are. The more positive the people around you will become. See, there's already potential for you to inspire others to be better and they'll hardly even notice you're doing it.

Some conventional wisdom I've read says 'positivity attracts positivity' but, I disagree in part. It attracts all sorts of reactions, so just be your best in each moment, in each situation. Imagine this and, yes, it's rather self-centred, try to imagine for every good thing you do, especially and specifically the stuff nobody else sees, that you are awarded 'life points' and I imagine you'd rather have plenty of those than just a few. Imagine those life points convert to the imprint you leave on this planet. While you're on it and even after you've gone. Feel good about what you do and if that's about making money, fine. If that's about being a great worker, that's fine too. If that's about being a great family member or friend, then brilliant. Whatever you do, make sure you feel good about it. Don't be left pretending about this one, ok!

This book isn't about trying to get you to change who you are, rather, I hope to simply help you to decide what it is you want to achieve and then help you to move in that direction and then stick to the job. It might be that you decide to change course some way down the line. Perfect, but don't bail, don't quit what it is that you strive to do and want to become.

It's ok to be flexible sometimes, but don't mistake flexibility for a chance to bail

So, what are you going to find here. Well, the basic premise is 'slow miles are better than no miles' (I'm not so much an 'it's the taking part that counts' kind of bloke). What's the difference you may well ask? I think there's a huge difference and it's all about the effort required to complete. Just taking part smacks of someone that started something and didn't finish it. I'm more about the getting the job done. We can't all be super-fast or super strong, mentally or physically, but we can be our best in whatever we do.

It's ok to tell everyone you're doing your best, or for that matter, people guessing you're doing and being your best. But, the final judgement to be made is more about you, convincing yourself, that you did well.

Taking part smacks of turning up and having a go regardless of the outcome. I think life is more about doing the preparation first, being at the start line ready and knowing that barring disasters or bad luck, that you'll complete! Please do away with the thought that I'm talking about a race, or a competition, or any kind of physical challenge, I'm not! This is me talking about life's challenges, whatever they may be, and the tenacity required to complete a task.

Think about that finishing moment, the completion of the goal, think of it as a red carpet with people that you don't know, applauding you. You'll be inspiring others, not expecting them to inspire you. Be a contributor to the positive energy pool of your world and those people in it.

Whatever made you buy this book, you can be the person you want to be, and the amazing news is, you took several huge steps by reading this far. Join me and my friends in here and be ready to be inspired to go out there and be the best version of you. Be ready to believe in yourself, because that's what it takes to improve. So much of what this is about is simple, trust me, it is.

You have just got to put in the effort and we can all do EFFORT!

Enough for now, except to say, I remember my school report was graded two ways. Work and Effort. God loves a trier they do say, so, in this book, let's not worry about talent too much, let's concern ourselves with graft, let's focus on agreeing to do the hard yards and then stick to it!

So, back to that question 'what makes this book different?'

Well, I've not read everything there is to read about motivational techniques, but we are all about going back to basics by extoling the virtues of hard work, not dwelling on what's happened before and, of course, taking things in manageable chunks, but, most importantly, I think, it's about helping you to rediscover the 'no fear' mentaility you had when you were young and that innate ability to just ''avago'. Whatever yesterday was about, today deserves your best of you!

Johann Wolfgang von Goethe

'Until one is committed, there is hesitancy, the chance to draw back, always ineffectiveness. Concerning all acts of initiative and creation, there is one elementary truth the ignorance of which kills countless ideas and splendid plans: that the moment one definitely commits oneself then providence moves too.

All sorts of things occur to help one that would never otherwise have occurred. A whole stream of events issues from the decision, raising in one's favour all manner of unforeseen incidents, meetings and material assistance which no man could have dreamed would have come his way.

Whatever you can do or dream you can do, begin it. Boldness has genius, power and magic in it. Begin it now'

I've read somewhere that this quote may have evolved somewhat since it was first written, had bits added to it that aren't attributable to Herr Goethe, but, you know what, I don't care. Howsoever it was created, I think it's a brilliant mantra for anyone and I'm giving it to you but ask only this, read and re-read, it's so much more than it might, at first, seem.

Learning to walk

Three times in my life, I have had to learn to walk. Two of those times has been to *re*-learn that very taken for granted skill, once, after a motor cycle accident and, a second time, after my knee was totally replaced. Here's a thing. My knee op has left me with a brute of a scar, starts way above my knee and finishes just below it. I was rather conscious of it for a while. I used to wear long cycle shorts for a long while after the operation to hide it. One summer's day, I was sitting in my studio in a pair of shorts and the scar was on full show. Ever keen to crack a joke in life me, when I was asked about the scar, I said I'd been attacked by a shark on holiday in Australia, my answer was believed and since then, I've always said the same thing, mostly, I'm called a big old liar but, occasionally I'm believed, phase two of the ruse, is to stretch the yarn and explain what a mess the shark was in after I'd duffed it up a bit, usually then, my cover is blown!

It is what it is, I make the best of what I've got.

So, learning to walk in adulthood…the first of those two occasions was easy, well, I say easy, the re-learning process started hours after the accident occurred. The second time, I wasn't allowed to, or even wanted to, start walking again for several days, too much pain apart from anything else.

Before I bore you too much though, what's my point?

My point here is simple, sometimes you must start over, sometimes you must go through a long, tedious and tough programme just to get back to base. Just to continue doing what you've always taken for granted. A

17

river, for example, is an irresistible thing, it will flow downhill, and nothing will stop it, but now and then a rock will get in the way. The river simply diverts to the side or around the rocks. If the rocks are high, then the river will pool and flood over the top, there's no stopping it, and whilst we aren't rivers with a never-ending supply of rainwater stocking up our supplies on high, my philosophy is that it's all about being a bit more river.

In 1976 after my near-death motor bike experience with the side of a Morris Marina at nearly 60mph, I had no choice but to get back on the merry go round and hang on. I was young, and it never occurred to me to slow down in my rehab; there was football and rugby to play, there were nights out and my apprenticeship to complete. Thirty years later, I refused to live with the pain in my knees any longer. I'd managed to get a promotion at work that included Bupa insurance cover, which allowed me to have not only a full knee replacement, but also after-care from some excellent people that gave me what can only be described as a new lease of life.

That all said, I look back now and think the me of today would have pushed even harder to get back to fitness and health, than the me of 2006, I left it a bit late and, as I will mention elsewhere in this book, it's one of my only real regrets in life. Getting one's head around the simple fact 'we are here for a good time not a long time' is a tough one and, in my generation, there's a few things you had to get as quickly as possible after you left school, a family, a house, a car and all sorts of 'things' that go along with them.

Possessions are important to me of course, but, as the years tick by, I crave experiences more, I get bored with 'things' sooner or later, but challenges and the experiences associated with doing them are, for me, far more important. I don't dwell too much on 'how wonderful it would've been to do some of things I do today, when all of me worked at its best' No point to this way of thinking… things are as they are, and that applies to you too, you can't change what's gone and you can't change what you did.

What's done, is done!

What you can affect, starting with your very next thought, is how your day goes, how your tomorrow goes and how those days that are immediate to you, shape the rest of your life. How the people around you are affected by your actions and how you might improve their life. Try not to analyse it too much, though, just take a leaf from the book 'The Secret', where the core message is being positive in everything you think, say and do.

Now, don't get me wrong, there will be times when negative shit goes down, of course, but every time you make a conscious thought about your plans, your intentions, your reactions, then at least try to make them, or some aspect of them, positive.

And hey, those 'leaders' amongst us, who can't stop spouting psychobabble get on my nerves, do they you? Some days, we just can't get that positive vibe going, I get that, but don't give up on it, if today isn't going to be a lottery winning kinda day, then keep your chin up and, like with everything, just do your best. It's easy to just take a time out, set the mind to positive mode, and at least make the next thing you say or do, have a positive slant to it.

The Secret tells us that trying to be positive at all times, brings you closer to positive things and positive people. Well, it's a great theory, but, sometimes, circumstances can be mighty persuasive to the contrary. I think it's better to say, 'do your best' and, like progressing from a 5k park run to a marathon, it's a time-consuming change that has no end date, just an end game goal. Most of us know the phrase 'baby steps', well, it works for me and I know it works for most people, because huge steps and short term huge goals can easily set you up to fail. And not the near miss kinda fail, but the 'what's the point' to this, downright negative mindset kinda fail. I tried all that, next Monday, I'm going to.................. '

Does that resonate with you?

So, a bit more about that week after my knee was replaced, and who am I to say, 'be like a river, dodge the rocks and keep going', it took me several days to get used to the Zimmer frame and hobbling with a stick. I had a mini break down I suppose you'd call it and called into question why I'd agreed to have the operation in the first place. That week, I suffered pain as bad as any pain I've ever felt and the early days of the rehab, especially the initial attempts to get mobility into my joint and that awful swelling control bag they used were just awful

I got into a place where work, home, family and friends were off the radar. Learning to walk again felt like I was in danger of not actually surviving, maybe being stranded in a hostile remote place might better describe it, but I felt like I was in the trenches and the objective of being able to walk pain free was my only objective in life.

I know what it's like to feel like that, really, I do!

Mine is not to try and tell you what to do, mine is to tell you what I did. Once I got home, I religiously followed the painful physio exercises I'd been given, after walking up and down the garden steps until I was in too much pain and had to stop, I'd wait for the pain to subside and then go do it again. Rain or shine, I was out in that garden, up and down, up and down.

Another week and I got my trusty old mountain bike off the wall of the garage brushed off the dust, pumped up the tyres and raised the seat so high I hardly had to bend my knee to rotate the pedals full circle. Up and down the cul-de-sac I'd go, each few hours an extra circuit, wobbling slowly up and down the road. A few days passed, and I dropped the saddle a half an inch and did even more reps despite the extra pain of that extra knee bend. Slowly and surely, the saddle went lower, the distances crept higher, the speed increased slightly and my reps in the garden increased. Between the two activities during the day, I was busy almost all the time.

General anaesthetic during the operation meant that several weeks passed before I could sit on the sofa for many minutes without falling asleep and, at night, I'd spend most of the dark hours awake with the throbbing pain in my knee. I was cautioned against doing too much by family and friends. I ignored the advice and stuck to the plan that my personal trainer had given me.

Evenings, I'd lie on the floor watching TV and put weights on my ankle to strengthen my quads with my foot painting invisible alphabets in the air, my heel hovering six inches above the ground.

Success was most evident during a follow up with my consultant, who called through to his secretary and boasted that I'd managed 120 degrees of bend in the knee - seemingly that was a first for any of his patients - that's my kind of result I thought!

And, I thought it was smart to return to work less than the 4 weeks that my initial sick note stipulated and promptly got kicked out of the office because it contravened company insurance rules. Sadly, that made me a bit happy too, because I was proud of the fact that I tried. I genuinely wanted to get back to work, get back into my routine and prove to the world that I was OK and ready to continue with life as normal.

Here's the thing, though (and I realise this is a little controversial but I'm going to have a swing for it), I am sure there might be some people whom it might suit to prolong a situation like this. Not everyone wants to get back to work and, sadly, it is the case that there are probably people who would exploit a situation that would involve staying off work, avoiding doing stuff and generally taking some time out of 'real life'.

Why mention it you might ask. Well, I've wagged off a few hours at work on the shop floor in my youth and I've been guilty of times when I've settled for far less than my best. My point is, why would you do that? Why waste time bunking off doing the hard yards, because once you've done those hard yards, the rewards are far greater than the 'feel-good' of chilling out excessively or even going at things half-heartedly.

Imagine if everyone, no matter how hard you work and play or how hard you work at avoiding doing your bit, gave an extra 5% towards being a better person, and by that I don't mean extra effort, I mean, making some sort of improvement in your contribution to the world, to people, to family and to friends.

Having to learn to walk again brings with it many opportunities and, to a point, I'm using my story as a metaphor for anyone's life. Just getting back to the previous status quo would be such a waste. Learning is amazing, and, the older I get, the more I realise every day is not just a school day, but every day is one where learning something new and indeed, trying something different, should be almost obligatory in your daily task list, including weekends!

This book is a testament to this approach, one which will try to persuade you that, whatever your starting point, and however bumpy the road ahead appears to be, your best is genuinely within reach. Lean that bit farther, try that bit harder, believe in your own tenacity and courage and you can 'learn to walk' again.

We have collected stories, anecdotes thoughts and reflections in the hope that, somewhere between the covers of the book, you might find the inspiration to be the best you can be, however limited and limiting your own circumstances might prove to be.

Don't just wish for it, work for it!

First Steps

It's OK telling everyone to face their fears and do it anyway. It's quite another thing to be faced with a task that one can't fathom out how to do! How to write a book, for instance? OK, I'll come back to that.

How to go about completing my first endurance challenge was easy, when, too many years ago, I agreed to take part in the UK Three Peaks Challenge. It's a 24-hour thing, well, more importantly, it's not a 24-hour thing, the general idea is that you finish it off in *less* than 24 hours and, back in the day, it was all about smashing the other teams that were taking part with you into oblivion by going faster and harder than they did. Organising that and going on to complete were, for me, relatively easy. For many people, this challenge would be a dream come true but, whilst every weekend throughout the summer, hundreds of people succeed and raise lots of much needed money for their chosen charities, it remains a challenge too far for most.

Each to their own, of course, we all have varying talents. In putting pen to paper, so to speak, I am simply taking the first step towards writing a book, it's a huge project and it would be easy for me to accept defeat before I've even got this far. I ask myself, who would want to read my stories, who is going to pay good money to listen to me, how do I make it happen? My goodness, it's a minefield!

I tried this several times and on one occasion I sent several sample chapters to around twenty book publishers, just a couple responded over the following few months, they all said no, the rest, didn't even do me the courtesy of a reply

So, what you do, is ask for help. And, regardless of your task, you will be amazed at how much help you'll get. In the book 'Feel the fear and do it anyway' Susan Jeffers famously points out 'When the pupil is ready, the teacher will appear'. Sometimes you must submit to such a theory and be patient. Trust that such a thing might happen, but maybe, just maybe, you must be on the lookout for that 'opportunity moment' as it flies towards you, it might smack you across the face and be so obvious, but, then again, it might be a little less assertive.

I like to think I'm one of life's fatalists, it's just how I am. Bold, some might say confident, in the main. Stubborn, oh yes, but I have my insecurities, that's for sure. I, like millions of other ordinary people, always thought I had a book in me, you, the reader, will be the judge of whether I'm right, or wrong, or maybe a little of each. I could grip you for a chapter or two, then lose you in chapter three If you're at all like me, in the countless books I've paid good money for, I get a bit bored when the reading gets a little heavy going and, before I know it, life's tendency nowadays to simply move on to the next thing has its way with me.

In this book, though, you can pick and choose. I'll introduce you to many ordinary folk, telling their own stories, of real times in their lives - actual events. You can read all the stories, hopefully you will, or just the ones that take your fancy, but the thread will be consistent throughout - feel the fear, but do it anyway.

25

A finish line can take many forms, and, sometimes, not making the finish line can be extremely rewarding and that's where I'll go at various points throughout the book, because I'm keen to stress that you should not be afraid if your challenge ends before the finish line, because the word 'failure' or, more importantly, the act of coming up short is very subjective. If you become better through the act of trying, or, you've done your best during your training period and then given of your very best on the day, you can begin to reap the rewards of taking on something that initially might seem impossible.

I imagine some of you just got your first subtle judder of a cliché, and yes, there's a lot of motivational stuff around these days. They preach 'Impossible is nothing!' or maybe 'Everything IS possible' and lots of other stuff, so I'll leave that stuff alone, because, it can be quite intimidating. Some words on a poster or plastered across the front of your mate's T shirt (the mate who runs five marathons in a week, or the mate who cycles John O'Groats to Lands' End in 4 days, or just came back from the Himalayas having climbed Everest) …well, you get what I'm saying. We all have buddies that are hardcore nutters and do stuff, that we couldn't ever do. That's fine, because you need to get comfortable with this simple fact, you are you, not them!

Remember, it's important to be yourself

The stories you will read in this book have many common themes, one of them is that 'being your best' is very personal indeed and, sure, I get really frustrated in day to day life, when I see people that I think can do better, settling for second best, settling for a less than 'all in, all guns blazing effort'. Though, my own arrogance sometimes astounds me, because those people are actually 'having a go' and, at the risk of promoting the theory, that 'It's the taking part that counts' I'm sure it's me that's in the wrong.

Taking part is fundamental and, slow miles, are indeed better than no miles, so please, cut me a little slack, I'm certainly not perfect and, in writing this book, I'm having a go, even though I am not, and nor will I ever be, the best writer in the world. The metaphor must be, so what, I want to do this and I'm having a go!

So, let me welcome you to The Avago Team, because you bought your membership card when you started reading this. We are both now part of an exclusive club. At the time of writing, there's no website, there's no Facebook page, there's no twitter handle, or, Instagram account, or, indeed, any social media so far.

All we have is the power of You, the power of Us, the power of Team.

I've always believed in the power of Team. I love football, I love rugby and cricket. Most team sports I've had a go at and I enjoyed taking part when I was younger. I now enjoy spectating, but it's important to clarify here, competitive sport, in my opinion, isn't all it's cracked up to be. I've learned, over the last decade, that, for many of us, competitive sport is an intimidating arena that can have some very negative consequences. Get the idea out of your head that a team must be involved in competition and install the brain app that promotes the theory of the team that is about people working hard for each other.

I won't try to explain my overall approach too much here, but, suffice it to say, my experiences with exercise, including a decade of leading Group Exercise to Music classes, have persuaded me that exercise, through whatever form of motivation, is the key to a healthy life. Exercise is vital in our lives and the chemical effect on our bodies is as important to longevity as say, good nutrition and even happiness.

OK, so what's the plan here? First, to enjoy the book, I don't expect you to get off the sofa right now and go climb a mountain, don't worry! I think you're going to enjoy the read, for sure. I think there's some cool stuff in here and I want to start by telling you about the 'me' of a decade ago. Why wouldn't I tell you, I'm a windswept and interesting person! Honestly, I'm like the Pied Piper of Hamlin, everybody wants to be like me, follow me and do the stuff I do. Of course, I'm just kidding, but, seriously, ten years ago, the me of today is a little ashamed of how I was, well, maybe ashamed is a bit strong, maybe disappointed is a better word. Yes, I'll settle for that.

I had a good job, I had a nice detached house, I drove a brand-new German car and ate out at some posh places every weekend. I dressed in expensive suits and wore some very fancy cuff links in my double cuff, Saville Row shirts. See, told you I was windswept and interesting.

I have omitted to say though just how overweight I was, how much pain I suffered in my knees through being overweight. For too many people, obesity is a disease that they are encouraged at every turn to ignore. TV is hammering us with adverts for food that isn't good for us, tempting us to spend countless hours on computer games that promote the 'restart game' mentality, where being less than perfect can be rectified by simply 'rebooting' and starting again...if only life were that simple! For now, commercialism knows no bounds. The UK, the Western world, the developed world is a very greedy and selfish place and, sadly, this shows no signs of abating.

There's so much more to life than money, fancy cars, cool clothes and lots of expensive possessions. There is, however, a lot of pressure that we all either have imposed on us, or are putting ourselves under to achieve those things. I wish I could tell the 'me' of ten to twenty years ago, about the me of today. A regret, maybe, but it's too late for all of us to have regrets. It's never, ever, too late to make changes, though, never!

So, why not start today, why not take a moment to apply the brakes to the machine that is your fast-paced life and have a think. What can I do to get a little closer to being the best I can be? Don't try to do it all at once, these things take a while, it took you all your life to get to exactly where you are today and if that voice in your head telling you to make changes is too often ignored, then maybe it's bothering you for a reason.

Come on, let's do this, we are Team Avago!

Ten Years Ago

Ten years ago, I find myself at the busy car park at Pen Y Pass in North Wales near Llanberis. It's a hive of activity and still very dark. We greet each other, Tim, Bill, Chalky and me as we get our kit together - boots, gaiters, wet weather gear, rucksacks, food and drink. We want for little and, for the most part, we are well equipped. Chalky has forgotten his hat, but it's September and a mild day, his waterproof jacket has a hood, it'll do.

We are off into the mountains to enjoy a day of high mountains and a bit of rock scrambling

We crack open a flask of coffee and the chatter continues unabated. It's been a while since I was out with these boys. Back in June, we'd been in the Pyrenees and enjoyed the total isolation that can only be found early in the summer in southern France. It had been too long and a crack at the Snowdon horseshoe, minus the intimidating Crib Goch arête, had been, we'd all agreed, eagerly anticipated

The light was improving slowly, and the time passed quickly and once coffee cups and flasks had been stowed, it was time to lock the cars and head off. Bill, from near Glasgow, had been staying with me, Tim and Chalky had travelled up from Bedford and Cambridge respectively. We worked for the same construction firm and held down good jobs, Chalky had been with us until a few years previously and had moved across to an IT supplier that I was working closely with.

Despite my anticipation, a tinge of guilt pricked me. I'd left France back in June with a plan to shed some weight so that I could enjoy my hill walking more. When I'd first walked with all these guys, I was always at the front, but around the time of our French trip, I'd struggled to keep my weight down and here I was, again, wishing I'd worked harder at my diet and exercise regime. Still, as ever, I'd have to do my best and see how things went.

The weather forecast was good for the day, windy and cool, but, best of all, dry. The craic was fierce; we had a lot to catch up on. Our employers, as ever, were the main subject of conversation and, of course, we four knew exactly what it would take to make everything right, make millions of pounds extra profit, and, in particular, pay us more and make our lives easier. We knew best, of course we did. I'm tongue in cheek here, to a point!

Back then, I was a regional manager in the south east of England, Tim, was, and still is, a planner. Bill did the same job as me in Scotland and Chalky was an IT systems trainer and programmer. We were all doing well for ourselves.

We cracked on up the wide, flat and easy track known as the Miner's Path. Dawn was in its full glory now and the light lifted our spirits further. Even though the car park had been busy, it was still early morning and it felt like we had the mountain to ourselves. Even on this flattish path, I was struggling to keep pace and contribute to the conversation. I worked hard to warm up and keep up, I bluffed taking a short break to 're-fasten' one of my laces, I knew all the tricks, anything but admit I was not as fit as I knew I should be.

We continued, and, as the incline steepened, the problem for me worsened, the boys just ahead of me now, chattering and laughing, me, at the back, doing my best to keep up.

The thoughts flying through my head were the same as always 'why can't I remember the struggle of this when I'm having an extra biscuit, or that second pint at the restaurant with my dinner, or seconds of pudding, or an extra sugar in my coffee', but, no, it doesn't work like that, out of sight, is very much out of mind. The exertion required to shift the extra five stones I was carrying was mostly evident when I was hill walking, which, sadly, wasn't often enough. Not often enough, because I loved spending time with these guys and not often enough because, frankly, I needed more exercise.

I toiled on, the next turn, the next slope, the next mile and, sadly, the first to suggest a break and sit down for a brew and a sandwich. Over the imposing Lliwedd cliffs, west bound towards Snowdon, the scrambling would take anyone's mind off just about anything, it was a delight to be there. Once finished, a steep slog towards the summit of Snowdon and the summit cafe awaited. Time for yet another break. My buddies were more than accommodating of me and we enjoyed the day as a team, but I knew that I was the one holding them up, and despite my new knee from two years before, I was feeling pain in both my knees, simply because they were having to work so hard to haul my bulk around the route. The hours passed, and Tim was always by my side, Will and Chalky busy in conversation about their families and happy chatting to each other as they strolled along. On more than one occasion as I winced stepping down onto uneven rocks and the angles jarred my joints, Tim would ask if I was OK. 'Of course mate, thanks' I'd bluff and blow my answers to deflect from the real issue - I'd become totally unfit. It was awful, it took this great day out to prove to me what a mess I was in.

In the past, I'd been round that course in a much quicker time. In the past, I'd always been at the front chivvying the others to get a move on. In the past, I'd be planning the next outing as we were descended back to the car park, but, today, I was embarrassed with myself, no, I think I actually hated myself!

We enjoyed a coffee in the cafe at the car park, with a piece of cake after we'd got changed at the finish. For sure, that day, I'd burned a few thousand calories and the cake had truly been earned. We chatted until it was time to leave, it had been a great day out and already, my travails had been forgotten.

Predictably, thoughts of a tasty dinner were in my mind - oh so quickly do the struggles of the mountains desert you, only to be replaced by the same behaviour that impelled you into the struggles in the first place. The mountains, God's own treadmills, are most unforgiving in that regard and, once you've left, they forgive and forget you all too easily, leaving you to return to the grind of the rat race, which, more often than not, takes no physical effort, and takes all the shortcuts when it comes to a healthy lifestyle.

After we arrived home, showers and a pot of freshly brewed coffee, the TV is on and we decide to order Chinese. Bill has stayed with us many times, but I'd never ordered from my favourite Chinese for him. China Paradise was about three miles away and usually prepared the food within the hour and, indeed, that night was no exception.

Soon, a hearty array of goodies festooned the table, a bottle of quality French wine I'd brought back from holiday and we ate like kings The walk was discussed and, as we both recalled some of the highlights of the day, my mood suddenly turned, and deviated sharply South. I felt a huge cloud come over me. The meal had almost been polished off, my first thought was 'I've earned that' and then the real reason for the gloom struck me. No, I'd not earned it, I'd eaten far more than I'd earned and felt so guilty, so weak and so annoyed that, despite the stark lesson of earlier, I'd seemingly learned nothing! What was I to do? I was brave enough to discuss it with Bill, and, as any sympathetic friend would, he told me how hard we'd worked and that I was being too hard on myself. I took a sip of the wine. What on earth could I do to stop this familiar cycle? What would make me take control and sort myself out?

The answer came out of the blue, 'Kilimanjaro'. I thought for about six seconds and then said it out-loud 'Kilimanjaro' and Bill sat back, swallowed a mouthful of wine and chuckled 'Aye, what of it?' he says.

We had talked about it a few years ago. What's stopping us I asked? 'Nothing' he replies and waits for me to respond. 'Exactly, nothing' I say. We stared at each other for a few minutes, I wanted it, he wanted it 'We could raise thousands of pounds for charity' I say. 'It'd be a blast' he says…Silence, both of us grinding it around in our heads, the sound of the cogs shifting was almost audible, though, ironically, the silence was deafening. I made my way into my study, left Bill at the table, booted up the computer and went back into the dining room, sat down, picked up my wine

Silence!

'What are we waiting for?' I asked.

'Nothing at all' he replies…

Silence!

A knowing glance and moments later we are on the PC. Twenty minutes later, we've paid our deposits for the following February, six months away - we are going to Africa! Six months away, the trip of a lifetime. Six months away and I've got the reason and the motivation to change everything. The cost alone will force me to make the changes I must make, to turn things around and make everything better.

Six months to reflect and understand, that the only day that counts is today and any mistakes I've made are in the past.

Tomorrow is another day and I can write a new chapter, but today is the day to commit to that change and plan my way forward. Tomorrow is exciting but today is even better. Once that trip had been booked, certainly for the foreseeable future, there would be no failed tomorrows, because I had to make every day count. I needed to lose that five stones, I needed to train hard and that in itself was a challenge. I'd need to find somewhere, a gym or health club with stair machines to allow me to do the specialist training. The positivity in my head was mind blowing, I was finally motivated, and it felt somehow different to all the false dawns I had experienced. At least I had to hope so, I had just slammed five hundred pounds on my credit card and, more to the point, I had to find another two thousand to pay for the entire trip and the kit I'd need to tackle the challenge properly.

This was it, as I fell asleep that night I hoped, but it was six months later that I know for sure, that I'd found the winning formula, the secret to regaining my health and, in the end, it was such a simple thing to do.

Preparing to Succeed

I was excited, that was the great thing, I was excited and, furthermore, I could see that the time-scale I'd given myself was achievable. 'Smart goals don't just apply to the workplace' I thought. Smart goals we got told, are the route to success at work, so why not in my private life?

Following on from my weekend with Bill and the impetuous decision making after the Chinese meal and the glass of wine that might have just been the difference between just another discussion and doing something meaningful, I had business meetings in Carlisle. As always, for me, this involved leaving early to escape the heavy traffic on the M6. Mid-afternoon, I hit the road south and drove straight to the David Lloyd complex close to the town centre near where I lived. Hands free (of course), I had called them from the car on the journey home and made an appointment for five o'clock and checked they had stair climbers in the gym. The gym membership would be my enabler, and I thought a decent venue like Lloyds would be a worthwhile investment, not least the great parking facilities so that I could train without worrying about my BMW getting damaged. Oh yes, I can remember being so very anxious about such things ten years ago, it makes me chuckle just thinking about it now - what a total waste of my time.

I was greeted at the reception by the Gym manager who apologised that he was going to be showing me round instead of a member of the sales team, they were all busy, but they wanted to make sure I had everything I needed to help make my decision about whether this place was for me. It was impressive, as was he, a semi-pro rugby league player for the Leigh Centurions. I was given the full guided tour and managed to dodge the normally obligatory gym induction session, it was perfect.

Two stair climbers, which he said were hardly used by anyone, countless rows of jogging machines and bikes. I get bored in gyms, never go near the weights, never use cross trainers, and usually avoid the running machines. In the past, I'd been to countless facilities like this one, mainly to play squash (which is another story, as is my football). But, let's just say, I'd found myself very much missing competitive sport and there was a big hole to fill when it all stopped.

I was taken for coffee and got to sample the social area, which was better than anything I'd ever seen before in any of the sports centres I'd been to. Big comfy chairs, lots of room, a Costa coffee, food bar and Sky Sports playing on the big flat screen TVs mounted all around the place. Cool tunes playing through the hi-fi system, it was plush!

I asked my guide if we could do the joining stuff and he went off to get someone from the sales team. Twenty minutes later, I'd joined as a racquets member and had full access to everything the place offered, including squash, which, despite my knee problems, I would be able to dabble in if the feeling grabbed me. The next stage was complete, the trip was booked, the means to the end had been now been arranged. I made my way back to the car, clutching my temporary membership card.

I drove home and smiled to myself because I'd sorted things so quickly and decided that the next evening would be my first training session. I'd try to keep it sensible for now, start as I meant to go on, decide on a programme day by day and then stick to it. No more long term crazy schedules that I would certainly mess up. I arrived home, and no sooner had I parked the car, than I grabbed hold of my dusty and trusty mountain bike. Before dinner, I'd go for a short ride up the hills, a cheeky little climb towards Winter Hill north of Bolton, which should give me something to aim for. The first time would be tough, but I was keen use the bike to help me get into shape for 'Kili'. I was into the house, changed and a bottle of water slammed into my bottle carrier on the bike, garage door closed, then a few laps of the cul de sac to remind myself how to use the gears (what I did learn was, it needed a service but, I could manage for now).

I cycled off towards the main road and the moderate hill at the end of my street that lasted only 100 yards had me blowing hard; not a great sign. I knew, though, that this was just the start. Onto the dual carriageway north and my next challenge was a complicated traffic light junction, which had me doing not a great job of the lane choices I needed to make, then left, into a half mile incline that forced me into bottom gear and forced my heart rate through the roof. I slowed my pedalling speed down a little. Back then, I knew nothing of cycling technique, cadence, posture, group sets and cleats, they were all alien to me. I'd bought the bike when I was in much better shape - the last time I'd been on it, I was sure things had seemed so much easier.

I slowed down even more, this was typical of me, I wanted to be like I was years before, without the hard work that it used to take to be in good shape. Football and squash were a thing of the past, but I knew cycling was perfect for my bad knees - low impact, and potentially high intensity. I didn't realise it at the time (but I would when I was sitting outside the Bob Smithy pub at the top of the ride that evening), that this time was different, I really was committed, and I really was going to climb Kilimanjaro in six months.

A short respite at the foot of 'Old Kiln' and then, gradually, the gradient steepened and, again, I was in cardiac arrest territory. I could see the hill stretching a half mile ahead of me, and, much as I wanted to maintain this progress, well, it just wasn't going to happen. The reality was very different, stately forward progress towards the top of the hill was the best I could do. By the time the give way sign appeared, not falling off was my only goal, and, eventually, blowing like a steam train that was ready for the knacker's yard, I climbed off the bike at the top road.

I climbed off and pushed my bike across the busy road to the pub. I was grateful for a chance to let my breathing settle back down, but it was taking its time. I was dripping in sweat and felt most uncomfortable. I sat in the smokers' porch that had recently been built outside the side entrance and marvelled at the view across Manchester and the Saddleworth moors and beyond that the Derbyshire hills and as far as the Berwyn hills in Wales. I was deep in the satisfaction of knowing that my journey was really under way, the path to the summit of Kilimanjaro was one that I could follow, if not see in its entirety right now. I was ready to take one step at a time, for once, to had a realistic plan.

Those early months flew by and I found myself hitting all my training goals. I never missed a single session. There was just enough pressure on me to do what was required. There was just enough time in my week to do this right. Three to four times a week, I was out on the mountain bike, my routes were getting longer each time, especially as I learned where all the best trails were to get me off the main roads and enjoy some tame off-roading. I was in the sports centre on at least three evening a week too and, previously, where I found every opportunity to have rest days away from the training, I was now looking for reasons to do my training more, rather than less.

Training sessions, on and off the bike, were getting longer, the stair climbers were horrendous at first but what didn't change was the pool of sweat I put down as the sessions got longer and longer. The sweat was now a result of long, hard, concerted efforts as opposed to a few minutes of pain, panting and sufferance. I was that lone figure on those unpopular machines, nearly every night. I'd cycle to the gym, do a session and then cycle home. Eventually, I was integrating both, and after training at the gym, I'd cycle up to Winter Hill on the way home.

My diet was improving every week, I'd decided not to go full stop on the 'dirty food', instead, I'd make incremental changes such as cutting out sugar in my coffee and then change nothing else for a week. Then, I'd cut out full fat milk and switch to semi-skimmed. Then, I started taking a one litre water bottle to work and filling it at least twice during the day. I was happy with the changes, my food got healthier almost by default and the weight was slowly, but surely, starting to come off me. At first, it took what seemed like an age to shift the first few pounds, but, by the November, I could see a difference almost every time I got on the scales.

My cycling got quicker, better and became fun. The stair climbers were becoming boring, in that I was on it for over an hour each time, the running machine sessions were an hour and the ride home was taking in even longer distances, and more metres of ascent. My clothes had been bagged up, literally in bin bags, and put in the loft and I'd treated myself to new clothes that actually fitted well, and by that, I mean I'd not waited until I was back in my preferred size. Instead, I bought stuff that fitted well and made me feel good. The entire programme was a joy to execute and every time the going got tough, I'd simply allow myself this fictional stroll towards, but never up to, the summit of Kili'. I had found the way to make this happen and every day I felt like I was a step closer to the goal. Every day felt like it had a part to play in the challenge. I had started fund raising on Just Giving and money for NSPCC was flooding in. We'd chosen the charity on purpose, it's a national charity that is held in great affection by just about everyone. Kilimanjaro is a few metres shy of 6000 metres high and so, our target was to raise £6000 and it was going well.

My home life benefited, my work benefited, I felt confident about my appearance for the first time in a very long time. I got compliments, all the time, and everyone helped me to work even harder. The usual

Christmas and New Year food challenges simply didn't materialise. I was far too focused on the plan and, better still, I was declining foods that were high calorie, I just had sensible amounts and kept to my hydration strategy.

I didn't need to get expensive coaching, so my gym membership was my only monetary cost. My time investment was a pleasure not a bind. Everything felt great and, best of all, simple tasks at work that somehow irritated me before were somehow put into context, there was suddenly more to life than work which involved driving huge distances around the UK and the trivial computer problems that came with my IT role.

By mid-January, I hit my target weight, with three weeks to spare. The training continued unabated!

One Sunday morning, in the New Year, I decided to do an early morning gym session. A first for me, it was just before 10:30 and, as I slid my membership card through the card reader, the music emanating from somewhere filled the corridor and, it seemed, the whole of the building. I walked along the corridor and pledged to see what was going on. A door with a porthole window seemed to be the source of the din and I peered through. There were orange and grey static gym bikes, the exact type of which I'd not seen before, almost like a racing bike on a frame, every bike was in use and everybody was drenched in sweat. I looked left at the front of the class and, on a raised plinth a woman was shouting above the music with the use of a head mounted mic set. The music was bouncing, and everyone was cycling to the beat of the music as she barked her instructions. It was very evident that everyone was having a great time.

I had discovered spinning and, what I genuinely hope is a lifelong passion.

What I also discovered at that point was the issue of what I'll call sustainability. I was lucky, spinning and the passion for cycling that took me over, has allowed me to maintain a high level of fitness to this day. And my German 'friend' Goethe's theory was right. By having a go, by being active, by constantly pushing myself, something positive ensued and I think it will always happen like that. It's just sometimes we neither build sustainability into our health regime or realise when it's happened.

Sure, when Kilimanjaro was finished in just a month or so, I'd be looking for more challenges because that was the mindset I was in, that is the mindset that you can have too, just by taking those little steps and always trying to be positive.

It might surprise you or you might be aware of it, or, you might plan it, but, howsoever you achieve it, it's about positivity and application. It will work. Go for it!

Fate and luck come into play when you push the boundaries. Don't wait for things to happen. Be in situations that will expose you to experiences that will change you for the better. Be amongst people that have that mentality. Don't be scared to get into that place, immerse yourself in it, be that person that creates exciting new horizons just by picking one new thing no matter how small.

I'd joined a gym to get fit for Kilimanjaro, but I really did not like the actual gym area and needed some specific machinery that would help me with my training. By being there, I found Group Exercise to Music - spinning initially but then other forms of group exercise.

I stop myself there, this is about you, not me, but does my thinking appeal to you? Apply your own specifics because you know what you enjoy doing. It's just, right now, that thing that you do enjoy may still be hidden to you. What will bring it to the fore? What will help you find the things that will help you be the healthiest version of you. You have your part to play in your future. And let me tell you, every shred of my being is shouting when I say, 'you are the main player' in your own life movie.

Take control, because you need to. Take control, because if you let others do so, then you'll live your life the way others want you to. Take control, because you deserve to enjoy the things that you want. It's that simple. If you don't, one day, you will regret it. So, why not start today with that idea or that wish that's been jangling away in your head.

The one thing I've learned of all things, is that every single one of us has dreams and hopes, most of which are within our grasp. Who knows what good stuff will happen when you change course, change direction in your map of life!

Looking back, that Sunday morning, and having applied

those principles, I not only found a brilliant way to enjoy
exercise that would stand the test of time, but I found
the core part of the business that was later to become
V1ntage Studio.

Kilimanjaro

The week before Bill and I set off for Tanzania, it was all about the trip, planning and packing, preparing and arranging. Work was a distraction, everything else was a distraction. Each day, my kit lists got a little longer, but I became happier that I wouldn't be short of anything or want for anything whilst away.

Not long after we'd booked the trip, we'd each received a letter from the travel company asking us which route up the mountain we preferred for the ascent, the letter also explained that we had to take American dollars to spend and hundreds more dollars to pay our temporary licence to be in the national park of Kilimanjaro. On arrival in Tanzania, a local agent had been appointed to look after us for the duration of our stay. At that stage, we had no preference, nor any idea how to make the decision about the route. Fortunately for us, my friend Tim had completed the climb a couple of years earlier, so he and I spoke at some length about his decision to opt for the trail called the Machame route and why he thought it was a good choice for us.

That done, I bought a book about the various routes up the mountain and could find no reason not to follow in Tim's footsteps.

The kit list included everything that a backpacking trip would require, plus a few pills and potions that had been recommended to us. Vaccinations, they said, would be expensive and comprehensive, all would have to be up to date and stamped to make sure we didn't fall foul of any aggressive illnesses. There had been much debate between us about pills and medication that might help us cope with altitude and whether we should take them. It was all quite compelling, and the many unknowns of this trip were making for a truly memorable experience even before we left.

By the morning of the drive to Heathrow, I was happy that I had everything. My trekking rucksack was rammed to the brim, it was effectively my suitcase and the weight was on the limit. I had another backpack that I would use as hand luggage on the plane and I would utilise it to carry all my valuables and the things I might need over the next 36 hours as we travelled to Africa.

To Africa! I could barely believe it, but yes, it was finally happening!

Bill picked me up on his way to Heathrow from Scotland. To be honest, we were like two schoolboys on their first trip away from home on their own. The conversation was constant the entire journey. We parked and headed into the terminal, all the usual behaviour in the airport, a coffee and peering into the screens to confirm our flight was going ahead as planned.

We headed towards flight check in. We were early, hours too early, but the long drive meant we had to build in some time in case of hold up and traffic problems. All to no avail, the journey had passed with no incident. We were behind a couple of people even though the check in gate hadn't opened. As the queue got longer, we chatted with the others and it became apparent that three of our party were now with us, Colin, Dave and Lee. One of them told us that they'd been informed that we five were the only people from my travel company that were travelling from the UK. One other person, who had been living in London up until recently, was already at the first lodge in Arusha awaiting our arrival, Anastasis Contoratas, a Greek banker, was the sixth person.

As the queue for check in lengthened, more and more trekkers that were heading to Kilimanjaro joined us. Remember it wasn't just our travel company that was sending Brits to Africa that day and I wondered, had they prepared as well as I had done, were they on the Machame route? It was exciting, I was impatient now to get through check in and then enjoy some time with my book, a coffee and my headphones. Enjoy some music, get calm for the long flight to Addis Ababa, then onto Tanzania via Entebbe.

As the wait began to grind a little, the calm banter turned into excitable chatter as a chap in a shirt and tie, with an airline badge on, appeared to be trying to explain something to the two guys in front of us at the head of the queue. I craned my neck and tried to hear what was going on and, as the airport official left, I settled for just asking the guys in front what was happening.

'The flight has been cancelled!' one of them said…

Over the next ten minutes, the two guys tried to explain to everyone that we were going to be taken to a hotel nearby and our flight was in fact not cancelled but had been changed to the next morning as our plane was in Rome, with a damaged windscreen and awaiting parts that would enable them to fly to Heathrow and turn the plane around. As the news settled in, the five of us discussed the developments in what could only be described as stunned astonishment. I was devastated.

What would this mean? I couldn't get my head around it. Our itinerary was crammed up until the last but one day, which was a rest day in Moshi. Did this mean our trip was off?

How could the people in Tanzania make up for the lost time?

How could I find out?

Everything was rather chaotic, and, frustratingly, that would continue to be the case for the coming hours.

Information was scant and none of us really knew what to do. It almost seemed more like rumour than fact, but the more we chatted amongst ourselves, the more it seemed that we would not be flying that day. I felt deflated and Bill clearly felt the same way. All I could think was that our itinerary dictated that a 24-hour flight delay wasn't possible, how could we still do all the things we'd been sold in the Kilimanjaro package, with one day less to do them in?

We both struggled to process the information.

Bill called the travel company, it was past five o'clock and nobody answered. He hung up.

'Answer phone' he says. I ask him 'was there an out of hours number given?' he shook his head 'didn't listen to it'. He called back, listened and wrote down a number. I called it and a woman answered, I explained what was happening. Seemingly, the airline staff were required to take care of us. I explained to her that the next 24 hours weren't really a worry to me so long as she could ensure all our connecting flights still worked, but I stressed to her that the time after our arrival in Tanzania was what concerned me, and I gave her the worst-case scenario that we arrive there only to find out that a one-day delay meant that we couldn't climb the mountain.

She tried to assure me that everything would be ok.

'Not really good enough' I said, I asked her to explain how it would work, in reality, at the other end in Africa. How could we fit a seven-day expedition into 6 days? It felt like I was getting somewhere then, and she agreed to discuss the problem with the agent in Tanzania and get back to me.

During the time I was on the phone, Bill had been given a voucher for a bus ride to a nearby hotel and we made our way out of the airport. Bill, Lee and Colin stuck close by, as they seemed at least as confused as I was about what was going to happen next.

The last hour or so had been happening alongside a rather humorous situation where a dozen Indiana Jones lookalikes had arrived at the queue for the check in. A larger than life, loud and rather eccentric Scottish man was making himself known to everyone heading for Kili. My tolerance of loud and overwhelming people is limited at the best of times and as he laughed off what was going on, my short fuse was getting even shorter. Nonetheless, he seemed to be in my face most of the time over the next few hours. His entourage, noisy and irritating, were becoming, quite frankly, a pain in the arse. On the bus, at the hotel, they seemed to be revelling in the fact that we had an unscheduled night in an airport hotel. It came to light soon that our rooms, our food and even our drinks were going to be free, I was guessing these boys were planning a bender at Ethiopian Airways' expense.

The very long queue at the reception desk in the hotel gradually receded and, fortunately, all our team were given separate rooms. It was now that Dave made himself known to us, our fifth team member, a Scot like Bill. We pledged to meet up after a shower and freshen up, to get some food and to get to know each other better.

My complete dissatisfaction with the situation was eased very slightly by the enormous double room I had to myself. I dumped all my bags in the corner, got undressed and took a refreshing shower. I towelled dry and checked my phone for the call from the travel company…nothing.

It did occur to me that it wasn't in the travel company's interest to clarify whether or not we would still have time enough to climb the mountain. Like most things, we worry most when we are lacking information and, usually, it's needlessly so. I relaxed on the bed, sent a text to Bill and asked if he'd heard anything, the reply came straight back in the negative. He was in the bar already with Colin, I decided to head down and join them.

Indiana Jones and his clones were already there and making plenty of noise. I ordered a drink and settled down with our team. Lee and Dave arrived soon after and we began to compare notes on the scant details we had. We agreed it was fair enough to assume our summit moment was in jeopardy and gave it till 9pm to call the emergency number again

Despite the situation, we got on famously. We talked about what had brought us to that moment and what each of us was expecting from the trip. Dave, a senior manager with Tesco and his dry sense of humour. Colin, an IT Brainiac from Brighton and Lee, a cheeky east-ender who worked in the city of London, we all got on really well and I was pleased with the mix. Fascinating really, but everyone shared one single thought, the fear of failure. Nobody said it, but it was there. All the talk was about high altitude (and what, for me, are myths) different ways of coping with being at 6000 metres above sea level, pills and potions. God willing, mindset was going to be my best, and probably only, tool!

We had some dinner and by 9pm I was ready for answers from the travel company. I was confident they would have positive news.

I made the call as the others listened intently. I was shocked when there was no news other than the fact that we could expect to be flying 24 hours late. Our flight was assured now. The representative had spoken to the airline and they were confident. What she couldn't confirm was how was the Tanzanian agent was going to cope with the delay and our expedition. This was more than annoying and, try hard as I could, there was now the prospect of having to try and get a night's sleep, not knowing how, or even if, our trek was going to be affected.

Sleep happened, it had been a long day and we all met again as agreed at 7:30 for breakfast. Nobody had any news and we agreed I would call the representative again after 9am. During the night, we'd been told via a note left under the door, that we had to be at the hotel entrance for 10am and that our flight had been brought forward to early afternoon. Things were looking up. I made the call just after 9, this time a man answered the phone. I made sure the news about the flight was passed on in case anyone else outside our party needed to know.

There was news. Our whole itinerary had been juggled and we would still be having a summit attempt, it would mean less time away from the mountain and mean our night in Moshi was cancelled, our rest day that had been scheduled for the day before our flight home had been cancelled too and we would have to walk straight off the mountain into the airport taxi.

I was over the moon, I couldn't have cared less about the rest day, and so I headed up to my plush room, re-packed my bags and made my way to the front of the hotel - time to get going!

The bus arrived, and all the hikers flooded on. Will and I grabbed seats and soon enough we were on our way, the short hop to the airport terminal, out of the bus and back to the familiar check in zone of the day before. Saturday was considerably busier than Friday, our check in desk was just one huge mass of people, it was hard to see where our queue needed to be, or if it had even started. There were bulging queues for other flights, people, cases, trolleys, bags, almost chaotic, but at least we knew we were on our way this time.

It didn't take too long to get through check-in and, before long, we were settled into the not so comfy plastic chairs of the main departure lounge with a take away coffee, my hand luggage and one of my eyes, and one of Will's eyes, on the screens all around us watching for our instructions to make our way to the gate. This too didn't take an eternity, and it was mid-afternoon before we knew it.

David, quite a solitary chap, sat himself down next to me, we started to chat and swap information about our jobs, hobbies and families. Tesco, it seemed, ran its own transport logistics company, of which he was a Director. Don't ask me why, but I was surprised when it became clear he lived not twenty miles from me in Blackburn. Two teenage children, second marriage and seemingly very happy.

A very tidy and orderly man, I remember his finger nails were as smart as I'd ever seen on a man and every time he took something out of his hand luggage, he'd smooth the pockets out and zip everything back up so as not to lose anything, I guess. His specs were either on his face or in the box, inside the hand luggage. He was keen to talk 'mountain kit', as was I in those days, and it turned into an interesting sparring session of who had the best of what.

I think Dave won. He won in more ways than one because he would research stuff and that meant he didn't impulse purchase. He'd bought all that gear having spent hour upon hour reading about it. I couldn't help but admire his knowledge of all things hiking, not least an extensive knowledge of the Munros in Scotland.

Now, for those of you that don't know about Munros and peak bagging, the Munros are a huge 'list' of mountains in Scotland, all of them are higher than three thousand feet, not only that, but strict rules apply to what is and what isn't a Munro. Dave took it upon himself to explain exactly and in some detail, what the elevation drop had to be on all sides of a Munro summit for it to be included on the list. Remind me to invite him into our tent if I'm struggling to get off to sleep, I thought to myself.

Bill was sitting on my left chuckling away, knowing the strict limits of my boredom threshold. I made my excuses and, whilst heading to the gents, took a leisurely wander back through the posh shops, Burberry, Watches of Switzerland, Mont Blanc etc. and looked through the windows and wondered, why on earth would anyone spend all that money on those things, in an airport?

I grabbed myself another coffee and braced myself for the long wait and maybe some more unsolicited information about mountain measurements. When I arrived back at our 'camp', Bill was chatting to Lee. I sat opposite them and sipped my coffee. Our Bill, always a great listener, and Lee, a very enthusiastic lad, who worked in the City and was doing rather well for himself it seemed. He enjoyed football and squash he boasted. I say boasted, everything he said, had a tinge of 'I'm better at this than you' kind of ring to it. He was good value though, and I decided once he'd calmed down a little, that we'd get on quite well. He had a boy racer car, a new house in the East End and showed us a picture of his girlfriend. He had to be back in work on the Monday after we landed in Heathrow on the Sunday come hell or high water and was already anxious that his employers would be less than delighted if he was late for work that day, or, God forbid absent. At this point, I'll cut him slack, I was that soldier, but not on day 2 of the trip.

Stressing over work could wait until the flight back at the earliest.

Colin joined us, Dave returned to the conversation and, happily, we really did get on rather well. Case of having to, maybe. Everyone was trying their best, and none of us knew what sleeping arrangements were going to be, so best get used to each other early on!

Colin, I very much liked. He was in IT like me, a good bit younger than me, maybe early twenties and a cracking sense of humour. He had just started going out with a Swedish girl he worked with and said just enough about her to persuade us she was almost all he could think about! He travelled all over Europe with his job and was clearly super excited about the Africa trip. We all were. And, as I finished my second coffee of the afternoon, Lee shouted out 'Gate 27 boys, we're off!'

Boarding and take off went without a hitch, we were bound for Addis Ababa, the plane was crammed. Bill and I settled into our books and, after a meal, calm descended on the cabin. I was reading a book about a famous cyclist, Lance Armstrong, who, back then, was best known for being a cancer survivor, seven times winner of the tour de France, head of the Livestrong charity and inspiration to many millions of people. I'd bought the book to read on the way to the summit and to try and help me sleep.

Strange really. Even if I'm enjoying a good read, sometimes reading was all I needed to send me off to sleep if I was restless. I was expecting the overnight camping to be uncomfortable and, unlike in later years when I finally decided to ask the doctor for a few sleeping pills for trips, I hadn't stumbled on a solution, but I was getting through the book at a canter, the story was gripping!

Mid evening now UK time, February, and outside the plane, pitch black as we headed south. The plane seemed to avoid any turbulence, it was a very comfortable flight.

Eventually, Addis Ababa and a long wait in the airport for us for our flight to Entebbe and a chance to stretch our legs. I always remember Addis Ababa in Ethiopia as the place where nobody had heard of queuing and, despite my best efforts to cope with this, I found myself taking the 'when in Rome' tactic to heart after only a very short while.

We never left the plane in Entebbe, but most of our fellow travellers did and, shortly after, as they shut the doors and we began to make our way to the runway, it was obvious that we had about 4 seats each on which to spread out and get some sleep!

It had been a long journey and we were on the last leg now, it was a short hop to Kilimanjaro airport and we landed safely, taxied to the small airport terminal, alighted via stairs to the tarmac a hundred yards from the building and walked across. It made me chuckle that we weren't herded like cattle into the building and nor did there seem to be any security as such.

It was hot, despite being late afternoon, the skies were pale grey, and the sun felt strong but was rather muted in the sky. It was very hot! There was less than fifty people getting off the plane. We did the admin. and a local man made himself known to us. The five of us gathered our kit and he ushered us to the car park, slung all our bags onto the roof of a long wheelbase land rover and we climbed in. He hadn't tied the bags down and I spent the first few miles looking backwards half expecting to see them bouncing off the tarmac, I must get a grip and relax, I thought.

The next leg of the journey was interesting. Large airborne insects came and went from the cabin of the old land rover causing us much hilarity, all shapes and, scarily, all sizes of bugs and weebies seemed to be taking an interest in us. Our driver seemed perpetually to be caught unaware by the brutal speed bumps every mile or so and had us hitting our heads on the roof, comical, but painful!

Mostly, we sat in silence and looked out of the windows, tired now, the long flight was taking its toll. Every inch of this long, straight, dusty main road was flanked with shanty buildings, people standing around everywhere. I'd been to Sri Lanka in 1992, which took me a little by surprise, but this was startling! Thousands of people every mile, walking, talking, standing and watching, nearly everyone turned to look as we drove by and, then, another speed bump would catch our driver, and us, unaware and have us all out of our seats. He drove just a little too quickly.

What struck me also, if not every dwelling, then nearly all of them, had satellite dishes, great big ones in many cases and, even more apparent, despite the obvious poverty (so many people were so very thin), were the number of people chatting away on mobile phones.

Less than an hour and we turned off the main road and started to wend our way along bendy roads, again, a little too quickly and we soon arrived at what appeared to be an ordinary house. We were asked to go in and a woman came out, saying "hello" in good English. The walls of the house had maps and pictures, there was a desk and some big packs of water. She asked each of us for the three hundred US dollars that we'd been told to bring, that would purchase our individual licences to allow us to be inside the Kilimanjaro park and to then climb the mountain.

It took just a few minutes and then we left, drove another ten minutes and swung in between a set of gates, up a steep hill and, in a cloud of dust, came to an abrupt halt at the entrance to a large place. We had arrived at the Karama Lodge. No words were spoken, we just got out of the truck and our luggage was passed down to us. A woman came from the main entrance and welcomed us to the Lodge, also, a guy strode across, it was our last but not least team member, the larger than life and handsome Anostosis Contoratas, he had a beaming smile. He'd been waiting nearly two days for us all to arrive, our team was now complete.

Into the main reception, which wasn't like any hotel I'd been to before, sparse and hollow, not very welcoming at all. One at a time we checked in and Bill, ahead of me, was given keys to our room. A man showed us to our place, on stilts but in amongst trees and shrubs, it felt like a real taste of Africa, very exciting!

Once inside the room, we were left alone to settle in for the night, dinner was being served at eight o'clock, we had a couple of hours. Both of us eyed up the shower in the corner of the room, well, I use the term 'shower', but it was more shower basin, shower head and a curtain that spanned the two walls in the corner of the room. There was no soap and no towels, thank goodness, we had brought both. 'You go first dude, knock yourself out' I said, and he gratefully accepted.

I lay on the bed, under the mosquito net, undressed and wrapped myself in a towel, there was no privacy. What there was though was plenty of big old flying insects and crawly things on the walls and ceilings. Small wildlife everywhere!

The shower started, Bill pulled the curtain and went in - silence. 'Just waiting for the water to warm up before I get under it' he says, and the moments ticked away. Soon it became apparent that there was no hot water. I looked around for a phone to call reception, no phone, shit!

Bill turned off the water, I offered to go to reception and ask them to deal with it. I did so but was told that someone had probably had a shower elsewhere in the hotel earlier and that the hot water had been used. I looked at him, waiting for him to offer an alternative, but no, that was it. There was no hot water on the complex for now, end of!

I headed back to our room, we laughed and put it down to being in Tanzania. My new-found tolerance surprised me, but it was obvious things were different here and there was nothing I'd be able to do to change it. What's more, I rather enjoyed this. In the space of 36 hours, the pace of life had dropped into a whole different culture, and it demanded we comply.

We used the shower to at least get a bit cleaner. Little did we know, that cold shower was quite literally a luxury compared to the facilities we would endure in the next week. We got dressed for dinner, chatting excitedly about the following day, our kit and what to wear, the weather and about how things might work, not least the big question of altitude and how we'd cope, it was the spectre of the trip.

I had learned something prior to leaving the airport, having always thought oxygen was in short supply at altitude and the higher you get, the less of it there is. Not true, for every one thousand metres of height you ascend, air pressure drops by roughly ten percent, so, we could easily expect breathing to be twice as hard as normal. What we didn't realise at that moment was that in our hotel, there and then, we were close to the same height as Ben Nevis back home and that we were gradually being introduced to the thinner air of Kilimanjaro.

We had a beer. Dinner was an odd collection of local food that left me hungry. The dessert was nice, though, and I made the mistake of having a coffee afterwards. Back at the room, sleep was a hard place to get to, but, eventually I dropped off and woke the next morning to my alarm, fascinated by the number of insects on the netting above my head. The room was in silence, Bill still asleep, his snoring usually kept me awake when we shared a room on trips before - he often told me I was actually the one keeping him awake. I looked around, above my head on the wall a lizard was hanging face down staring at me. About six inches long, I made to sit up and it scuttled off into the rafters of the building where the daylight began to appear between the walls and the sloping roof.

It was a pleasant morning, certainly not hot and no way humid, which I'd expected it would be. Bill was disturbed by my movements, I was running the water in the sink and he stirred. We exchanged pleasantries and were soon heading across for our breakfast, again, basic and none too tasty, the main plus was hot coffee and it was strong too. The milk was a bit odd, but I am always grateful for coffee.

We didn't have long until it was time for us to make our way to the main gates of the lodge about four hundred metres away. Not sure what to expect, we were all there ahead of the appointed time.

Staz, as our Greek friend liked to be called, fitted into the group quickly and easily, we all sat roadside and waited beyond the time we'd been given, soon though, the guy from the land rover appeared in a medium size coach with a couple of new faces, Samuel and Emmanuel were our guides, they were smiling and helpful to us as we again launched our kit onto the roof. We all had the bag which had been our hand luggage on the plane that doubled as our rest day bag. That was supposed to be staying with the local agent, but it seemed the impact of the flight delay meant this was coming with us on the trek, at least as far as the Machame Gate start point.

There were already others on the coach. We took our seats, most of the windows were open and inside the coach it was warm, the seats rather hard but not as hard as the suspension on the bus, or, the lack of suspension, I should say. Our route took us along more dusty roads for about an hour and, as the road narrowed and steepened, the roadside was teeming with people. Our coach stopped, and Samuel pointed to a guy who threw a bag up top and climbed on the bumper of the coach, hung on and thumped the window. Off we went again. The men roadside were now two deep and more in places, we stopped again, although the bus was moving very slowly now, another man joined the crew and hung off the back of the bus, we all looked at each other, Lee said 'Our porters maybe?'

And so, it was. Slowly, in a queue of rickety old coaches, we idled our way uphill, the heat was becoming increasingly uncomfortable and inside the bus, we were cooking! What struck me was the hundreds, maybe thousands of men looking for portering work by the roadside. It was another stark lesson of the difference between the western world I lived in and this, developing world reality. Work was hard to come by and our porters were clearly very happy to have been given a few days' worth of it.

I remember at this point how the books I'd read about the Kilimanjaro treks suggested we, as visitors, should be vigilant of our tour company using boys and older men to porter for us. I'd read stories of groups passing porters who'd collapsed by the path up high from heat exhaustion from carrying heavy rucksacks and equipment and our part in reporting our guides if they employed people at risk. Our guys all seemed fit and healthy and gave me no cause for concern at this stage

The Machame Gate was reached and though we were in a line of buses, the queue of vehicles behind us was

64

longer by some distance than that in front. We were ushered off the bus and our bags were passed down to us. This was it, the start of the actual walk.

We quickly got out of the sun and it seemed we were lucky to have a small shelter all to ourselves. David was speaking with Sam and came across to us and said we should brace ourselves for a bit of a wait as they sorted our paperwork. We chatted about the grim prospect of this being the last proper toilets before we hit the hotel prior to flying home in six days' time. Bill headed across and said, 'I'm going to try and have my last comfy sit down before we go'. Well, those were not his exact words, but it's close enough.

He came back, shaking his head 'I hope the wait you said we would have allows me to have another go'. I knew what he meant, no sooner would those toilets be out of sight than, knowing me, I'd want to use them. Well, I had nothing to worry about, I trundled across and it was mission accomplished a few minutes later. The toilet paper reminded me of the toilets at Station Road, Swinton Rugby League from the late nineteen sixties but, from what I'd heard, the 'thunder boxes' on the trail would make this feel like five-star luxury. Truth be told, the prospect of those portable toilets had bothered me more than anything else about the trip and I was not looking forward to using a 'thunder-box'.

An hour or so passed and it was beyond noon when it seemed it was time to leave. Our leader, Sam, gathered us and asked us to get our day packs on our backs. He asked only one thing, - to stay behind him on the relatively flat section that was the start and until we reached our first overnight camp. That seemed fair enough to me, he looked very fit and strong and we may well struggle to keep up with him, added to which, he was about to start the walk in shorts, T shirt and trainers. Little did I know, apart from a very battered jacket,that was all he had, a few T shirts, one pair of shorts and one pair of long pants, no boots and no hats.

Sam set off and, at first, it was like a test to see who could walk the slowest. We bunched behind him shuffling along the path and off into the even hotter, humid, jungle. No breeze, but, thankfully, only occasional glimpses of direct sunlight. It was baking hot, but almost felt damp. We trudged slowly, and, despite almost no effort, I was drenched in sweat. It didn't seem that long before Bill signalled that he was going to pull over and use the 'toilet', a good idea I thought. I did likewise, and Sam signalled a drink stop, which forced everyone to take out their bottles and hydrate. Our porters came steaming through at such a pace, I'd swear some of them were carrying their own body weight and more and yet, they were flying. It became apparent later why they had to move at such high speed towards camp one.

I couldn't have hoped for a nicer bunch of guys to climb Kili with - no egos, not really, Lee was a bit too keen to up the pace, but, as the youngest member of the team, I could understand his impatience. Everything I'd read, seen on TV and heard from others, especially from my friend Tim, was about pace and patience, I'd followed closely on TV a programme about the trek along the Machame a few months earlier, a week long programme, that followed a team very similar to ours, across their own Kili week, and out of the eight of them, it was the two youngest in the team that had fallen foul of altitude sickness.

Our day was a series of short strolls and drink stops, we noshed on our own personal stock of food treats, but we knew today was only a few kilometres and that, just beyond the jungle, was camp one.

We arrived late afternoon and saw the camp on some flattish ground, off to the right of a small building, well, a shack really, that sold cold drinks and sweets. Dark inside, not much to choose from, but the cold Fanta was a tasty treat, the guy took my dollars. As the size of the camp dawned on us, I, for one, was staggered by the sheer number of people that were heading up with us.

Now, I could see why our porters had to get here so quickly. Flat ground was at a premium and whilst there were two major local tour companies, seemingly taking up most of the decent ground and with their own portable toilets, we seemed to have been lucky or maybe our man Samuel was a more wiley operator than was at first obvious.

Emmanuel, the number two guide, showed Bill and I to our tent. We stowed our day sacks at the entrance, our main rucksacks were neatly laid inside, on top of the rather shabby looking mattress. Our tour information packs that we'd received months earlier had said the mattresses were 50mm thick, but, this clearly wasn't the case, although, once they might have been I'd grant you. I slung my big rucksack out the front and lay on the mattress, Bill did the same and we laughed together. It was real now, this was it, we were at the end of the first day of our Kilimanjaro challenge, I'd slept on harder ground than this when I'd been wild camping, and I was quite happy so far.

We got called to a rickety table and the six of us sat around as instructed and waited. Our camp boss, Henry, brought a steaming pot of tea and a huge bowl of popcorn. The milk in the jug for the tea was again, a bit of an odd taste, but I quite enjoyed this. It cooled a little, not much but enough to stop me from sweating while I sat still doing nothing. The inside of the tent had been stifling hot and the mattress had a musty smell to it. No matter, I'd thought, I have my micro pillow, sleeping bag liner and super warm sleeping bag - we'd been told the night time was really cold.

Dinner soon followed, it was good and before I forget to mention it, this guide company did decent food the whole week - we were in for some tasty treats. No beer or alcohol, but a choice of coffee or hot chocolate after our starter of soup and then the main meal of chicken and rice, one thing was for sure, my appetite was sated well and truly as I settled into the tent that evening.

Bill and I chatted for a while, there was no privacy on that camp and the excited chatter continued for hours. There was a noticeable increase in the excitement and people were calling out to look out of the tents, which we did. The sun was setting, blazing red and orange behind Mount Meru in the distance and oh my, what a sight it was. Slowly but surely the colours faded, and we settled back into the tent. We'd witnessed a sunset as good as any you might see anywhere in the world - vibrant, bold and quite spectacular! I thought there and then, that sunset was, by itself, almost worth the money we'd paid to be there!

Sleep was hard to come by and that first night was a long one. I couldn't even bear the thought of getting in the sleeping bag, it was so warm. Bill, as I was expecting, was snoring, but then I knew I snored in my sleep too, so I might get him back soon enough. I did manage rest for sure and, despite our long journey, I was disappointed with how much sleep I lost that night. As it turned out, though, day two wasn't very taxing and after our wakeup call from Henry and a warm bowl of water for a face and hand wash at the entrance to the tent, we enjoyed strong, hot coffee, cereals with tepid milk, and toast and preserves. It did make me wonder how on earth our porters managed to get all their gear this far.

There were more porters than us by nearly two to one. Despite a blur of activity around us as the porters struck camp, our breakfast table and chairs were left until last and we took our time about getting on the trail. Samuel left us as he and Emanuel and another guide finished their food. There were occasional hand signals from Samuel to the porters who worked tirelessly as they all moved away from the camp and left us contemplating putting on our boots and looking to Samuel for the way ahead.

Day two was very different to day one in only one respect, no shade from the sun and all of us were soon wearing our floppy hats, neck buffs and various pale coloured outfits to combat the direct and strong sunlight. It was only eight o'clock but already very hot. Nonetheless, a gentle breeze accompanied us on our way.

Drink stops, food stops and the barren, dusty, trails prevailed the whole day, a very gentle impression of height gain but almost imperceptible if I'm honest. So far, fitness wise, it'd been easy. Camp two, and the tea and popcorn that had been eagerly anticipated all day. Otherwise, and in every respect, it was a replica of camp one, right through the night, broken sleep, tossing and turning on the mattress, again, I lay on, rather than in, the sleeping bag, it was simply too warm.

The time for breakfast at camp two eventually arrived, heralded by the bowl of warm water for washing and then another decent breakfast, not least the hot strong coffee which I drank eagerly. The porters were soon striking camp around us, but gave us no impression that we were holding them up, nor that we had to rush. Again, we were on the trail well before nine o'clock, except this time the porters left after us and easily burned us off in the first hour, leaving us and all the other trekkers for dust. Each group of porters filtered past us carrying huge weights on their backs, piled high and, yes, every time I saw my dude, I felt bad that he was loaded to the gunnels and full with my entire trip equipment. In fairness, a lot of it should have been staying in storage at the hotel we failed to stay at in Arusha and we'd had no chance to lighten the load, short of throwing things away.

We arrived at camp three mid-afternoon after another day of dusty, hot, and parched trails. It was slightly cooler than previous camps but still a warm evening. Tea and popcorn was had sitting around our rickety table and even the flies seemed less annoying that night. We'd gained height this day and I felt strong after

what felt like our most productive day. We had earned
our food and our tea and popcorn had never tasted so
good

What was a little scary was I began to feel the growing
urge to use the' thunder-box'. It is almost ridiculous to
say, but I'd hoped I'd get back to civilisation without
having to use one of them, but, sadly, I was very much
mistaken. After we'd settled into the tent for a pre-dinner
rest and nap, the need was too much, and I gave in to
the box of thunder. I strode over with my toilet paper and
went into the empty one of two, wow, it stank! It was
disgusting, but it afforded me a little privacy and just far
enough away from the camp that I could do the needful.
Oh boy, what a relief! And, a decent thigh work out too,
being so anal (excuse the pun) about getting good
clearance between my 'pantage' and so on, the need to
get the job done and dusted was accelerated by the
burn in my thighs and calves as I tried to maintain my
balance throughout the operation.

Dinner was enjoyed, and afterwards Bill and I got out
the Frisbee that had travelled with us to many UK
mountains and the Pyrenees. We hadn't bargained for
the huge crowd of porters that congregated, fascinated,
around us. We threw it to and fro and Colin and Lee
joined in. We hadn't bargained for the interest that it
caused amongst the hundreds of porters and, soon, it
seemed we had an audience that included just about all
the locals. Some of them wanted to have a go and after
the first guy threw it so hard and nearly garrotted one of
his mates, we decided it might be best to call it a day.

The evening ended with us lying in the tent and me
reading more about Lance Armstrong, in the hopes that

it would make me feel sleepy. It did, and I fell asleep
with the book open in front of me. Sadly, only for an
hour or so, then the usual battle to sleep again, whilst at
the same time feeling wide awake. It was cold outside
as the first few hours of darkness turned to pitch black.
Bill needed the loo and came back from the trip beaming
that he'd also conquered the dreaded thunder-box.

It seems hard to believe the heat those tents retain, but
as he dawdled to get back into the tent, take off his
boots and zip up the entrances, the place got very cold
and I had to get into the sleeping bag despite still
wearing shorts and a t shirt. As the hours slowly passed,
I became increasingly aware of the cold and, slowly, so
slowly, eventually, as daylight started to dawn and the
sounds of Henry setting things up confirmed it was OK
to start getting ready, I decided to open the zip and poke
my head out.

What greeted me was a great surprise. Each tent was
surrounded by what to all intents and purpose looked
like mini snow drifts. The big rocks scattered around the
place, the same, as if a movie production company had
been through and made it look like winter in the camp.
The temperature though, was no illusion, it was freezing
cold. In less than two hours, breakfast eaten, every
trace of the wintry scene had disappeared as the sun
beamed down on our world and very quickly warmed us
through.

The breakfast drill was the same as the previous days,
except, I definitely felt a little short of breath. I stood to
eat my breakfast, and, for the first time, I had on my
fleece jacket. As always, the porters were busy striking

camp around us and, as always, we were left to take our time over getting ready.

Today, we saw the biggest Blackbirds on the planet, and we also saw the weirdest trees, which when leaned against, almost fell over as the shallow roots struggled to hold firm. Today, I read about how Lance Armstrong won his seventh Tour de France. Today I was inspired and today I reinforced that I was, regardless of anything, going to the very top of this mountain. Today, we arrived at a place called the Lava Tower and here and for the first time I was struggling to breath, plus I'd developed a slight headache. For good reason it seemed. We were at 4600 metres above sea level. Yes, the gentle acclimatisation was working, and we'd gradually made our way up to this point with very little noticeable change, but now there was no avoiding it, air pressure was down to half its normal level.

We ate our lunch here, although breakfast didn't seem that long ago. I took my first two headache tablets to try and alleviate the increasing thumping in my head. It was a constant nuisance now as I sat on the rock eating my food. Nothing to take my mind off the pain, we all were feeling it and the mood was increasingly sombre, despite the elation of each of us, reaching the highest point we'd ever been to.

The views were decent but, to be honest, the satisfaction I took from the place was the success of reaching 4600 metres under my own steam. Lee was coping, but was clearly struggling. Fair play, though, after lunch, he just got up and got on with it, quiet the most part, as was Bill now, both had gone into themselves to try and keep up. Colin and David were together as we started to drop towards our overnight camp at the Barranco Wall, Staz and me, getting to know each other, all seemed to be lifted as our headaches dissipated as the altitude dropped.

A couple of hours later, we walked into Barranco Camp, which was very hot and very crowded. Many of the teams had left the previous camp after us, but had arrived here before us as we'd taken a different, higher, route to this fourth overnight stop. It was sweltering hot and, as we clambered across boulders into our own area, the Barranco wall loomed ever larger with every stride towards it. It was an impressive and imposing cliff face that had us all standing and staring in awe.

Our guides did nothing to allay our fears of the ascent of the wall the next morning and it looked impenetrable from where we stood. Tea and popcorn duly consumed, we sat looking at it and debating where the path might go. Sure, we could see the entry point and that was pretty much it, the rest seemed hidden, or, as is so often the case with steep scrambles, there were so many alternatives that none had suffered so much erosion that it could be seen. The wall was the sole focus of our evening. We did pull out the Frisbee, but found it to be hard going, as the ground was so rocky and uneven. As the dark and dusk came over us, the view between Barranco and another high cliff to our right, afforded us a view all the way down to Moshi and the pinprick lights of the town looking so many miles away, but less than 20.

Sleep was only an occasional companion that night and not much more.

Surprisingly, the next day, despite lack of sleep, I felt good. After breakfast and striking camp, I couldn't wait to get into the wall, which, in the end, took less than an hour to breach and was something of an anti-climax. I could tell you it was more difficult than it was and at well over 3000 metres or if you googled a picture of it, you'd probably believe me, I've even heard of people that have been up it and said it was tough, but, I would disagree. Even so, it was a more interesting hour than any so far on Kili, but, of course, once atop the cliffs, the familiar dull headache returned - time to pop a couple of paracetamol.

Dusty, hot and very dry, today we were going to cover the same ground as we would've done over two days had we not been delayed at the airport. A late morning lunch was taken at what would have been night camp 5, but, as we were still making up time, we pressed on up steep trails for the rest of the day. We arrived at our final night camp of the ascent a little after 4pm, the heat was still quite uncomfortable, but no sooner had we stopped and had our customary tea and popcorn, than the rather stiff wind was telling me to get inside the tent which, unfortunately, afforded us a little warmth.

The wind became much stronger and, very quickly, it buffeted us, so we came back out of the tents to discuss the day. Dinner was served early and we had to stay behind in the large mess tent after dinner for Samuel to brief us on the next 24 hours. Half an hour later, we made our way to the tents and, as he'd warned, as the wind picked up and the sun dropped down behind the hill, we begin to feel the cold.

And so it was, by early evening, we were in layer upon layer of clothing and into our sleeping bags to keep warm. The temperature dropped dramatically and quickly. I'd never experienced such a contrast hour on hour as this. We had to try and get some sleep. Breakfast was later that evening at 11pm, yes 11 at night and we would start our push for the summit at midnight prompt. As the whole camp began to quieten down, Colin came to our tent to explain that Lee was in trouble. Nothing specific, but Colin felt that there was a chance he wouldn't even get started later that night.

I felt I had no part to play in that. We needed our rest and I told Colin I thought they should rest and try to sleep. Samuel came by our tent and asked if I'd take the back of the group with Staz, when we set off later, because we were the fastest and strongest of the six. I was quite proud of that and happy that my training had set me apart from the others alongside a young man who had just finished his national service, less than half my age.

Sleep took me, for a little while. I woke, and my head was freezing cold and there was the now constant headache. I was needing a pee, but tried to get comfy as it was past nine o'clock. I put on my fourth layer above my waist, a second fleece to try and get warm. Outside, the wind was noisy, and the tent was being blown around, but at least it seemed to still be dry. Sleep took me again and, before I knew it, Henry was rousing us and offering us the familiar pan of warm water to freshen up. Breakfast was ready he said, but we could eat it in the tent if we wanted.

We ate, we drank. I popped three paras.

It was time. Fully clothed already, we stepped out of the tent. It was absolutely freezing cold. The wind was blowing hard and we struggled to communicate. We stood waiting. What's happening? Why aren't we moving, I was so cold. We looked at each other, Bill, me, Colin, Staz. We looked at David; "where's Lee?"

It was Lee that was struggling to get moving.

Five minutes, six, seven. Soon I had to ask Samuel if it was OK to go back into the tent, but then suddenly Lee appeared. Colin told us he'd been sick during the night and the delay was because he'd been sick as soon as he ate his food minutes earlier. The guides had encouraged him to try and get something down, which eventually he had, only to throw up almost immediately.

He said he felt OK to try and summit and, moments later, Samuel was at the front followed by Lee and then the rest of us in line. Ahead of us, a stunning sight. Several hundred head torches strung out in a haphazard line ahead, maybe a mile into the distance. I looked at my watch, it was twenty past midnight. I was irritated by this, we'd been told we had to be away by midnight to ensure we saw the dawn from the summit. The gap between Sam and the next walker, was about three hundred metres, we it seemed, were the last team and by some way.

Head down, I kept myself to myself, I was vexed, but kept telling myself Lee was ill, kept telling myself, it could be me. In the thin air, though, my headache and the situation were really vexing me. Head down, keep going, head down, be patient.

An hour later, we had caught the last team, another half hour, we'd almost got to the front. A short break, drink, nibble some biscuits. Another half hour, we are at the front and moving well, my mood lifts. Another hour passes, and we take another break, I'm standing by a wall, having taken a few mouthfuls of food and some drink, the wind is cutting through me. I have never known it so cold, ever, but again, I thank God that it's dry.

Suddenly, a commotion beside me, I turn, I'm covered in sick down my left leg, we are all stunned and likewise the others too are covered in sick! Lee is crouched over and, as the minutes tick by, nobody able to talk, what becomes clear is that he's going no further. Samuel takes the time to explain to each of us, shouting into our ears to overcome the din of the wind, that Lee will be taken down by one of the guides and that meant he and Emmanuel would take us the rest of the way, but suddenly there was a huge caveat over us. One more person drops out and our challenge is over!

It is against the law for one guide to walk with several walkers, one to one, yes, two to several yes, but one to several, no! We said our goodbyes to Lee, told him to make sure he got down safe and wished him well, and now, we were at the back of the line again. The half hour stop had left me shivering and desperate to move on to get warmer. All worries over anyone else dropping out completely left my head. It wasn't going to happen, Will, Colin, Staz and David were all strong and fit guys.

We started to make ground on the silent, trudging, walkers. Higher and higher, the sound of boots shuffling against the fine grit on the endless zig zags up the mountain will stay with me all my life and, still, we are passing people. It seems to me like we are getting slower but, compared to most of the other teams, we are flying.

A break, a drink, a mouthful of biscuit and onward, the bitter cold biting my skin across every square millimetre. My headache now is really hurting my head and I pledge to swallow more pills before we finish our next break.

We stop, I chug the pills, there's no escape from the wind cutting through me.

We walk, heads down, in silence, the noise around us is deafening!

Another break, a sip, I can't eat anything, I'm done with food. Everyone is struggling now, the steep and relentless zig zag path is taking its toll and then, out of the blue, Dave shouts over the noise of the wind, 'I'm done, I can't stand this cold anymore, I need to go down'

I am, to say the least, stunned. He was so matter of fact about it right there, right then, at just a few hundred metres of ascent to Gilmans Point.

I take a moment to consider what he's just said and replay in my head Sam's words after Lee is taken back down. If this is true, we are done. Kilimanjaro will have defeated us. Well, for me, I thought, that's not happening.

I turned to Dave and asked him 'You're just cold right?'

'Yes' he replies, 'I've never felt so cold, ever, I've had enough mate'

I look at him, this has to change, I decide. In my rucksack, I have a lightweight jacket. I take off my pack, reach in and that's pretty much all that's in there. I hadn't planned to bring the jacket, but left it in as we ate our evening breakfast earlier, left it in, with my drink bottle and snacks to stop things from bouncing around, to fill the bag I guess.

I take off my Goretex, four season winter coat and hand it to him, 'here, get this on, you're going to be fine mate' I tell him. I reckon from his demeanour that he's already decided he's heading down and he smiles at me, 'thanks, it's OK'.

'No mate, it's not OK, at least try another half hour for me, with the extra coat on, let's see how you get on yeah!' my tone is less of a question that the words here might depict. I was determined he wasn't going to throw away this soon to be enjoyed success.

He pulled the coat off me with my help and I swiftly replaced my heavy winter coat with the flimsy wind-proof layer, which didn't seem to make any difference at first. I was frozen through, this was not pleasant at all. I looked to Sam, I was bossing things a bit now, 'Get that jacket on you dude and on you go' I gestured, it's time to smash this, I thought, and I was determined to keep Dave going no matter what.

Fifteen minutes later, things had settled, which was more than could be said for the fearsome gale blowing, dry but vicious from our right, incessant and strong enough that occasionally it managed to break our stride, buffeting us and causing us to stumble. The coat incident had us about a third of the way back in the long drawn out line of walkers, all heads down and silent, trying hard to cope with the wind.

On and on we slowly strode, passing other walkers now, slowly but surely, we got back into the groove and, as if Sam and I were in silent agreement about the need to push on, the stops ceased, and we just kept on going, heads down, wind seemingly going straight through us, onward, upward, slowly, but very surely higher and higher, the zig zags never ending.

Finally, as with all mountains, there is a top, well, in this case we hit Gilman's first, about one kilometre from the summit. Samuel explained where we were and explained that one kilometre and the gentlest of inclines was between us and the summit goal. One kilometre, but Bill looked like a man who'd downed ten pints of strong beer, he was leaning against me, in what seemed like an altitude induced semi-conscious state. His eyes wide and distant, Samuel told him to hang on to his rucksack and he would pull him to the top, if he wanted to go.

The wind was dropping now, it was calming down so quickly it hardly seemed real. Bill, propped against Sam, Colin and Dave, stood motionless and all seemed, at this point, keen to just get it over. Staz and I, with Emmanuel, seemed lucid enough, my head was pounding, and I felt light headed, but, at the same time, super elated to be so close to the top. Walkers were passing us, one by one, so slowly, everyone trudging towards the rim of the crater and now, the vast glacier perma-ice was to our left - on we went.

We passed many of the walkers and were soon at the front. It wasn't fast, it wasn't slow, it was, though, as if we walked in robot mode, one step at a time, the crater of the volcano to our right, deep and impressive, not really able to take it in. The wind had dropped to a breeze, the light was dawning quickly now and the scraping of boots on the floor, the trudge and grind to the top continued. It was then that we saw the Indiana Jones group, their leader spark out on a wheeled stretcher, he was almost unconscious, what on earth were they doing? But, as quickly as their plight was in my thoughts, it was gone again, and I looked round, Colin, Staz, Emmanuel, all behind me, Samuel with Will, hanging on for all he was worth, not far behind.

I wasn't proud of the state Bill appeared to be in, but he'd made it clear, despite the mess he was in, he wanted this summit!

On we went, lighter and brighter, the change in the view was startling. The bright orange glow, the day was dawning and into view came the famous tangle of wood that was the summit Uhuru Peak, 5895 metres, we were here! We had made it, the highest point in Africa, the highest point I'd ever walked to and my best ever physical achievement. Bizarrely, we'd brought the Frisbee, it was in Bill's rucksack - and that was where it stayed!

I had two jobs to do, I stationed myself in front of the wood pile, gestured Bill across, Sam brought him over and he propped himself on me, peering at Sam who took our picture on the camera that had been in my chest pocket to stop the batteries from freezing. We were shifted off the summit point quite quickly and, one by one, people arrived to get their summit pictures done. My second task was yet to be completed

The summit is bare, there are no stones, I asked for some time to myself, it was granted. I asked if I could walk away from the summit, away from the path we'd just come up, permission was given, but I mustn't stray too far. Samuel and Emmanuel were too busy with Bill, he was in a distressed state and needed to rest they said, I had the time.

It now somehow felt like I was watching a movie with these guys in it and I was at peace by myself, almost alone and elated, each sound amplified around me in my head, but voices were muffled and distant, it was truly, and quite literally, surreal.

I wandered about four hundred metres away and stood watching the summit scene. Emotions…emotions began to well up, I was choked now, and all I could do was think about my amazing Grandfather, William Henry Price, who'd been taken from me at the age of 71. No age, but so ill with, lung cancer and emphysema. His last year or so, a constant companion was his oxygen bottle and the mask. I found a few tiny stones, walked some more steps, a few more and gathered them together. This far from the summit, I was hopeful that they'd never be disturbed. I made a small cairn out of maybe a dozen small stones, which I truly hope is still there, as a tribute to him, from me. I was sobbing uncontrollably now, I was so proud of what we'd done, what I'd achieved, crying and smiling at the same time.

I looked up, the sun was up now, and the view was quite remarkable, the view was worth every penny the trip had cost. It was worthy of all my efforts and I don't think I'll ever see a better view, anywhere. Then it struck me, I could see the curve of the planet, yes, it was noticeable, left to right, it was real, and I saw it, once and never since, with the ground under my feet. I was looking at hundreds, maybe thousands, of miles of Africa and the curve of our planet. Now my tears stopped, and I smiled, the broadest of grins. I'd done it and, I'd done it with energy to spare.

Samuel was waving animatedly, I headed back. All we had to do now was descend more than four thousand metres in less than eight hours! Onward…

The Tour De Mont Blanc July 2017

So, let's fast forward nearly a decade.

It's approaching midnight, some six hours earlier, I'd been enjoying the summit of the Grand Saint Bernard col, the frontier between Switzerland and Italy, the clear blue skies and blazing sunshine had been made tolerable by the cool air of the 2500 metre altitude and the adrenalin rush of having climbed it under my own steam under trying circumstances. Six hours ago, I'd not been even slightly affected by the solitude of the moment, or that I'd been left solo by nearly all the support available to me, left to fend for myself on the frightening Tour du Mont Blanc, supposedly, and aptly, nicknamed 'the toughest one-day cycle race in the world'. A mixture of visual, scenic, stimulation generated a moment I'd never forget, a mental picture that was committed to my long term hard drive, the relief of having finished the biggest climb of this epic challenge. In my head, I was on the return leg, in my head I could enjoy the descent into the Italian town of Aosta, through countless picturesque villages and along mile upon mile of easy riding, which I'd earned on the thirty-kilometre slog to the Swiss, Italian, border that Italians call the San Bernardino.

Descending high Alpine mountains in excess of fifty miles per hour on a bicycle, is hard to describe, but let me try. The weather is perfect, the roads are dry, and the traffic becomes irrelevant because I can easily keep up with cars as they head down the road, in fact, sometimes it's me who must be patient and wait for the car driver to negotiate the twists and turns of the road, in particular the hairpins that threaten to catch you out.

There is a heightened sense of a caution, a need to be completely alert to the dangers presented every millisecond, the thousands, possibly millions, of sub-conscious decisions you make as you pick your precise line into each bend and then, out of the bend to gain maximum speed, safely, into the next long straight. At one point, I felt I was going faster than ever, later, my trip computer tells me I'd hit over seventy miles per hour at one point. It's a feeling like no other, I promise you!

Five and a half hours earlier, on that descent, I'd felt like I could ride all day, and all night, if I had to. Five and a half hours earlier, my bike was behaving perfectly, I had plenty of drinks, food and money on board. Five hours earlier, my loved ones knew I was safe and, five hours earlier, my life was totally and completely in the moment, I wanted for nothing other than to keep moving forward.

The scenery slowly changes into the urban sprawl that is Aosta, the temperature was climbing and every kilometre or so, I was reaching for my drinks bottles, it felt safe, I'd be able to get drinks before my stocks became dangerously low. I was coping with lack of support and for once, felt I was completely self-sufficient. The heat and cloudless sky, coupled with the effort of having to ride the bike, to have to put effort, considerable effort, through the pedals, I found my perfect cadence for the terrain. I was flying, low on my dropped handle bars, the discomfort of my narrow saddle was almost forgotten, still, I was in the moment and totally in the zone.

Let me take a moment to tell you about those rare moments in my life, where I've been completely in the moment, no distractions, and enjoyed complete calm and, to some extent, complete satisfaction with my circumstances. This state of mind is not exclusive to extreme physical exercise, of course, nor is it necessarily about 'happiness', whatever we might mean by that. But, for me at least, this state of mind comes about through a combination of working so hard, at something you are being your best at, that you're happy you've giving your best, when nobody is there to judge your performance apart from you. You may be so completely engrossed in your efforts that time passes more quickly than you want it to, because you may be struggling. But, and this is the crux, you will be struggling in the best way, suffering such that you reap rewards from it. For me, struggling and suffering when I'm cycling deliver such rich rewards and part of my aim with this book is to describe this well enough that you will seek this level of effort when you work out or exert yourself, in whatever way you enjoy. I must be clear, I do not think of struggle or suffering as negative things, and to add more foundation to that statement, the challenge described in this chapter has finally taught me that failure, if indeed that is the right word, is simply a sometimes-necessary step towards success.

Five hours earlier on that flattish road out of Aosta, which lasted for many miles, I was in a great place. In this state of being in the moment, on reflection and as I write, I know this has something to do with two of the big climbs I'd completed earlier in the ride, and how those climbs had caused me to suffer cramp, the like of which I'd never had on the bike before. It caused me to curse out loud, when there was nobody around to hear me, so painful that I'd ridden in standing position for maybe a quarter of mile or so, on multiple occasions to shake it off, and at least once, grasped a rock face to steady myself as I stretched my left knee joint, in an attempt to get rid of it. Had ridden through all that to a point where I felt I'd earned the right to be in the moment.

And, as I enjoy that memory while I write, let me also allude to the 'broom wagon', the French guy in the sweep van, the grim reaper as I nicknamed him for most of the day, the Grim Sweeper as he later became known. Every elite cycling race or event, like the Tour De France, has a broom wagon. In a nutshell, for the back markers, as in golf, which calls it 'making the cut', a point at which stragglers have to be told, you're not going to make the grade this time. In the case of the Tour du Mont Blanc, we had 19 hours to complete 330 kilometres and 8000 metres of ascent. Given the extent of the challenge, and the fact that my three teammates and I felt very much out of our depth, we knew from the day we paid our entry fee, that we were in this to do our very best, maybe complete the course, and maybe, just maybe, complete the course inside the 19-hour cut off point which was in Les Saisies, France. Despite the threat from the Grim Sweeper, I had been so perfectly positioned on my bike, my foot angle was perfect and my grasp of the bars, just right, I'd set the front and rear gears to the perfect combination for the flat road and had set my cadence, pedalling rate, to the perfect level, so that my heart rate was at the perfect percentage for just such a section of the ride.

The moment coincided with a unique event for me.

Five hours before that moment, a few hundred metres south of La Salle, on the busy bypass, I was signalled into the lay-by by the Grim Sweeper, who'd passed me a few miles ago, and in that place also, was my friend and the feed station vehicle with the organisers standing by, waiting for me. The moment I'd dreaded all day had arrived, I'd kept myself a hairs breadth ahead of the Grim Sweeper and now it was time to face the music. I was taken out of the race, there and then, my race number taken from me in one hand whilst they handed me dry, cold pasta, hot fizzy coke and some fruit pastilles, it struck me as, quite literally, a bitter sweet moment. I'd spent the day, battling against time, battling against the progress of the Grim Sweeper and his transit van with the yellow broom sticking out the top and the big sign on the back, 'cycling event, please be patient'.

The Grim Sweeper was a kind man, he had a job to do and maybe I'd escaped being kicked out at the previous station due to his patience, never mind the other motorists passing our event being patient of him dawdling along, mile after mile behind yours truly. He had been a kind man when passing me water through the window of his van as I struggled to keep myself hydrated five hours before that moment, in the dark and in the cold. In the dark and the sub-zero temperatures of the Col Petit San Bernard.

My friend's words, were barely audible, but the meaning wasn't hitting me, then, another of my friends appeared, they were both talking to me, with five hours to go until that moment in the freezing cold, both talking to me explaining why they themselves had pulled out - thirty degrees heat, twelve hours already, exhaustion and fatigue, levels of effort up those climbs that none of us had ever encountered before, a quite different, all new, level (welcome to the world of the elite cyclist). But I was not really hearing what they were saying, as I explained my determination to continue, regardless of having no race number and no further support, such as it had been thus far.

Five hours earlier, I'd carried on from Le Salle regardless, because I was in the moment so deep that there was only one option - to continue.

Continue even though I knew the Grim Sweeper was going to be taking away the road signs as he made his way back to the start/finish. My friend's misfortune became my ally, as I happily accepted the offer of his now redundant Garmin GPS, regardless of how much battery life it had left, it would help me navigate the correct route for at least a few more miles and in the spirit of the day, in the spirit of being in the moment, I'd worry about having to navigate by actual map and my event route card only when it was necessary. And, in that moment of bullish enthusiasm, I threw my leg back over the bike, clipped by left cleat into the pedal, pushed off, waved them all goodbye, safe in the knowledge that my friends would make good their promise…'You stubborn old dog, we will come and get you if you're in trouble!'

Five hours earlier, could not be more different than the midnight moment, however, in the pitch-black dark with both my lights flickering into oblivion and my hands shivering as I tried to get on my gloves. I was talking to a cyclist who'd shared the last few miles of the climb with me, and God forgive me, I so very much wanted him to stop talking to me!

After countless false summits on that climb up the Petit San Bernard, I'd finally worked out I could only continue by taking short rests off the bike, my own theory of climbing was in shreds. As many of my friends know when I'm hill walking or cycling, given the usual reserves of energy, I'd always rather keep going, drop the pace a little and keep going, I call it 'active recovery'. Well, this was a different place, I was empty, I was close to finished, I was allowing negative thoughts to rule my actions now. I think I was done. I ground to a halt on the ten percent gradient, as the light was dying, and the temperature was dropping fast, I waited until the road rounded a hairpin, to give myself a better chance of clipping my cleats back into the pedal when it was time to set off again. I sank onto my handlebars and reached behind me into my back pocket for the phone, told them back at base I was close to making the fateful decision, "I'll call you back at the summit of the col after I've eaten some food and assessed my situation". I desperately wanted to eat and take a proper rest while the food replenished me so that I could complete the challenge, there was still a chance, if only I could fuel myself.

The cyclist who had originally introduced himself as a polish scientist pulled alongside, it was almost completely dark now and our lights had been on a while now. 'Can I help you?' he asked. I was able to continue and so thanked him and we rode on together, my pace was painfully slow by now. Conversation was almost impossible, but my cardio levels weren't the problem, it was such a mental effort to just talk, but his enthusiasm for the place and his willingness to help me, was infectious and despite him having cycled a similar distance to me that day, his spirits were better than mine.

When we had met originally, we'd talked about bikes and gears and cols and the Alps, and the Italian Dolomites and the Pyrenees, he could see I was in a dark place and yet his eagerness to help made me feel better, despite the effort it was taking to talk. Twenty minutes earlier, however, I had simply ignored him, stopped my bike and got off. I genuinely thought I'd got to the summit. I leaned against the wall of a house, the house that indicated to me in my slightly delusional state, the house that was on the col, and took some cold breaths down, he'd slowly carried on and as I starred ahead, though, and I realised, yet again, that the mountain had fooled me into thinking the col summit was breached. Ten minutes before that moment, I finally got moving again after managing to get some fluids down my neck, pure nectar, every drop. My back bottle was almost pure water now, my tasty Robinson's juice flavoured Italian spring water in my front bottle had become impossible to drink, all I could manage was the free stuff. Five minutes before that moment, I put my head down and reset the gears, pedalled onward again and set my sights on the dark shapes coming into view as the skyline revealed what most certainly was the summit of the col Petit San Bernard

And now, this was the moment of truth!

In the space of six hours, the Tour De Mont Blanc had picked me up, lifted my spirits as high as any challenge I'd ever done and then slammed me into complete submission. In six hours I'd been through the full range of emotions, including, and, not least, the mind games.

Those false summits take their toll and the mountain gives no mercy, none whatsoever, there's no quarter given, nothing. And, metre by metre, it had broken me. Broken me to the point where quitting seemed the only option. Broken me to a point where quitting was OK, even for me.

The pitch blackness, as I hunted round in vain for the water that my team mates had left for me, the cold that was biting into me had taken me by surprise and indeed, had taken my fellow cyclist by surprise. His original plan to camp in his simple bivvy bag and micro sleeping bag was no longer an option for him - 'I will follow you down the mountain, we will ride together, it is too cold by far' he said.

As I stood in peace and quiet trying to eat some white chocolate, I was seeing things in the dark that I knew weren't quite real, it took several minutes to find my back up lights and with that paltry light, I could make out that the frame of the building in front of my emergency LED lights was real but, as I slowly swung round, my imagination told me the shapes were first one thing and then, as I looked again, something else completely. I turned to the other cyclist and felt I needed to tell him that my race was done and then he could start to focus entirely on his own safety – I had realised that I could only take care of myself. This realisation, and the hard, white, chocolate, were, together, proving a hard mouthful to swallow. I sipped my water, I chewed some more. As I stood still, it seemed to become increasingly cold by the minute. The fact was, I was no longer moving, but was simply shaking and shivering in the gloom.

My companion had done whatever it was that he was
doing and appeared to be ready to ride off. I offered him
several blocks of the white chocolate. 'All for me?' he
exclaimed, seemingly delighted and grateful in equal
measures, again I gestured the packet towards him and
he took the chocolate, smiling, eagerly chewing and
swallowing it down with much glee. As he left, I
wrestled with my emotions, and it took me several
minutes to finally decide what I was going to do. I'd been
cycling for some seventeen hours and whatever I
decided to do, it necessarily involved coasting down the
mountain to the next town or village, whatever that was,
and trying to warm up. I've descended many alpine
routes this last two years and I know very well, that
doing so has little to do with getting warm and more to
do with getting colder and increasingly fatigued. The act
of simply rolling down a hill takes no effort pedalling
wise, but every other aspect of descending in freezing
cold conditions is tough. It needs the rider to be on the
brakes, almost the entire time, it requires complete
concentration. It requires patience and time, and,
preferably, daylight.

So, my decision was made, I'd done my last climb for
today, I'd broken my last bead of sweat, cramp, wouldn't
trouble me again, and the feeling of relief was immense.
I could manage a short ride to the valley below, I could
do that and keep busy and maybe get a bit warmer.
What I didn't realise at that point, however, was what a
stark contrast the reality of that descent would prove to
be.

I think it took almost ten minutes to complete a basic,
thirty second task. Just to take off my gloves, to get the

phone out of my pocket without dropping it onto the hard floor beneath me, dial my friend's number without my glasses on and make the call and let my people know I was finished and I'd meet them in the town, in the valley below, the name of which they'd have to check for me as I was too cold to search on my phone for it.

Such a struggle! Such an infuriating and ridiculous struggle. Even colder now, I pull on the gloves, trying to compose my crazy breathing - an unwelcome companion I struggled to shake off throughout the whole of the descent and for some time after.

Short of breath and wondering how long this was going to take, I'd committed now to cycling to the town to be rescued off the course. I rolled onto the main road again and the incline was sufficient to quickly cause me to gather speed and require me to instantly hit the brakes.

My Polish friend was behind me, his headlight shining ahead, casting long shadows ahead of me, the gentle rush of the wind across my ears meant I soon lost him, not realising that my plight was made tougher because the LED lighting was all I had. I was alone and all I had to navigate my way were the intermittent white lines in the centre of the road. I was comforted by the vast expanse of sulphur yellow street lighting down in the valley. It looked quite close, which meant the descent would be hard on my arms and fingers, right then though, all I thought was, 'it'll not take me long to get down, not that far, can see the street lights, 'aint nothing, off we go, I'll soon be warm and safe in our car" and as I swung slowly around the first hairpin, a signpost comes into view and I can just make out Bourg St Maurice 31 kilometres. To be honest, I think I'm losing touch with reality a little, what with the crazy breathing and the white dotted lines in the road, it's all I can do to keep rolling safely and progress downwards

I was stunned by that sign, 31 kilometres still to go, surely not?

It's so cold, it's so dark, already my arms are painful. What seems like hours pass. Several times, the crazy breathing is brought under control, several times, my complete attention and focus is swallowed up by the white lines, which occasionally kick savagely left into 180-degree hairpins and cause my heart to race out of control for several minutes after each scary incident. I have no idea what's at the edge of either side of the road.

And then, the first car on the other side, the driver doesn't even bother to dip the headlights, I'm blinded. He flies past and I bring the bike to an almost standstill as I struggle to regain my night vision such as it is. I decide to stop the bike, compose myself, give my arms a rest, a rest for a moment and then onward, down and down, the crazy breathing, compose myself, white lines, another hairpin, another car, dipped headlights this time, takes me less time to regain my sight, onward and down. Slowly, each hairpin I see the Polish cyclist back up the hill slowly making his was down, but he's falling back all the time, I catch myself thinking 'wow, this is taking him forever and I can't go any slower than this anyway'

Crazy breathing, compose, focus and white lines, more cars, temporary blindness and more of the same, the sulphur lights of the town, they aren't getting any closer, it seems like an age and I'm still really, really cold. The crazy breathing is getting harder to control and then, a sign looms into view, mind games begin, I can make out three words and a number, I tell myself 'please, let it be single figure kilometres, let me be close to done with this.

The sulphur lights look no closer than when I set off from the top, another hairpin, another car, caution! The sign reads Bourg St Maurice 23 kilometres. I am distraught!

Less than a third of the way down! I slow down, I stop the bike, a rest for my arms which are so very painful now. Compose and try to calm the crazy, crazy breathing, which, if I could see myself doing this, I'd be inclined to think was being done for effect. No sooner have I set off and begun the battle of the descent again, my phone rings, imagine, cold hands, repeat the process back at the top, I miss the call, hell, I'm still trying to stop the bike when the ringing stops, a text follows, it's my provider telling me I've got a text. Phone out of back pocket, I return the call, it's my people 'We're on our way to Bourg St Maurice, take care, we will get there as soon as we can'.

Phone away, gloves back on, I'm glad of the rest for my arms, and off I go. I happen upon a small village, busy, people here and there, bars and restaurants, ski village doing its summer thing. It gave me such a lift just to be able to see where I was going and to see folk at their leisure. It gave me a lift because it gave me the sense that I was getting closer to the valley floor, cars, houses, street lights. However, as quickly as the village had come upon me, it was gone, and I was back into darkness again, breaking hard at bends, down and down, crazy breathing, compose yourself!

Another sign. 'Bourg St Maurice 14 kilometres' nearly two thirds now, another few cars, a few street lights followed, then darkness. More cars, the gaps in my crazy breathing seem a bit more relaxed now, in my head, I'm nearly done, the next sign tells me its 7 kilometres to go, more street lights, houses with the glow of their lights and reading lamps, people getting ready for bed, people in bed, down and down I go.

I feel such relief, street lights now, more than the gaps of darkness in between, the temperature is noticeably less hostile, the conditions feel less like winter now and suddenly, I'm on the edge of town, the sign says one kilometre to go. I feel like crying, the bike picks up speed, I brake hard after resting my arms for a moment, the speed had suddenly increased and needed me to act, it wasn't quite over, down and down, I allow the bike to pick up speed by releasing the brakes. Finally, I'm not out of control just by letting go of the brakes, relax, people, cars passing me without blinding me, the emotion of it all is intense, I roll past bars and restaurants, there are people everywhere, not one single person even looks at me. Surely, they know I'm so happy to see them and soon my people will be here, my chest heaves a few times and emotions well up.

I'm safe, I'm down, it's just a matter of finding a place to wait. I see a bus station, maybe I can use the toilet, I need to go badly, but it's nothing, the battle to get down is over, I'm OK!

In the moment, I've been in the moment for hours, complete focus and complete concentration, I am truly exhausted and I realise the extent of my decision. I've quit a challenge, for the first time in over 20 years. I know, I did the right thing, nobody made me stop, nobody will blame me for stopping, because I got right to the edge of my limit and that descent represented me teetering uncertainly on the very edge of my personal, on that day, extreme point. It felt surreal yet rewarding, I felt whole and completely satisfied, all in the same moment. It was over, regardless of the long journey back in the car, I had made it with only 29 miles and 1000 metres of ascent remaining, of completing this monster challenge. I had done, without any question in my own mind, my absolute best.

Thoughts from Team Avago

Kelly Stott

It's difficult to know where to start when I try to explain why, what and how my life has changed since 2011. But, I will do my best.

Initially, I just wanted to lose weight – fitness and health hadn't even entered my head. My partner of 21 years had asked me to marry him and I knew that I didn't want to spend our special day feeling self-conscious and huge, as I did every other day. The real kick up the backside was when I was having a discussion with my Mum about my weight and she said 'well, you could do with losing a good 4 stone'. I've always been able to count on my Mum to tell it how it is and, thankfully, her words had the desired effect!

Around this time, I received an email from a colleague telling me about a new gym that had opened close to my office where they were doing Zumba classes - would I like to go? The thought of going to a gym made me feel scared and uncomfortable. The thought of walking into a room full of strangers not to mention jumping up and down in my over 16 stone size body made me feel sick to the stomach, but I knew that I had to take that first step.

And I did!

Anybody who attends a place like my gym knows how important it is to enjoy the place your go to exercise and how life changing it can be for the people that really want to be there and change their lifestyle. Very soon, it becomes more than just a place to exercise. The support and friendship are second to none and, thankfully, this is what inspired me to continue my journey to improve *me*.

Before I knew it, I was agreeing to attend classes that I never thought I could do, spinning, circuits, padbox and Kombat (a mixed martial arts style class) to mention a few, as well as signing up to challenges. How did that happen?

At first, it really was just about losing weight, but the more classes I did, the more I realised how unhealthy and unfit I was. Following discussions with staff at the Gym, we came up with a plan, unbeknown to me, one of many plans that I would be working to in the future!

I managed to lose 2 stone by the time that my wedding day arrived in April 2012. Physically, I felt great and, mentally, well, I had begun to like myself. Being overweight isn't just a physical thing for me, it has a negative effect on me mentally. Taking that first step enabled me to enjoy my wedding day without constantly worrying about how big I looked and what people were thinking.

What next? That was the question I was asked when I came back to the gym after my honeymoon.

There had been numerous discussions about cycling events and, having not been on a bike for over 20 years, it was something that I wanted to avoid. This wasn't an option! An outdoor cycling session was organised for members who may not have been on a bike for a while but wanted to ease themselves into cycling. The session was fantastic, and I couldn't believe how much I enjoyed being on a bike. Before I knew it, I had signed up for the

Bolton Bash event, a cycling sportive that involves a long route of 60 miles and the short route of 35 miles, both very hilly. To my amazement, I completed the short route and have now done the event 3 times – improving on my time at each outing.

As well as cycling, I found another passion - the love of walking. I remember the day I made the decision to do the National Three Peaks 24-hour challenge. Some of the gym gang had gone off to climb Ben Nevis and I was following their progress on Facebook. I don't know what happened that day, but something stirred inside me and I felt totally inspired. Reading their posts, the sense of achievement and the support that they had for one another was incredible. I wanted to do it, so I texted the gym owner the next day. There was no going back now he said, 'once it's said, it's a commitment'.

We did many training walks including climbing Helvellyn and Skiddaw in the Lake District and Snowdon in North Wales. To say that I was scared is an understatement; I was worried that my fear of heights and failing would create a real barrier to me completing the challenges. I needn't have worried. The support that was given at each event was amazing and most certainly built my confidence. The gym people instilled into me a belief that I could complete any challenge and I soaked this up and got on with whatever lay ahead.

Team Three Peaks 24-hour Challenge ended up being just 3 of us and our driver Andrew – myself, Gareth (friend, Leader and Instructor who has his very own version of motivation that *works*) and another good friend Jackie, who you'll read about later in this book. We completed the challenge in 23 hours 12 minutes, the training paid off! I was so pleased and emotional; I will never forget it and it will always be an extremely special memory for me.

That question popped up again - what next? There had been mention of Total Warrior, seriously, Total Warrior, me! After a discussion with Gareth and a few of the other members, we got a group together. Warrior t shirts were made up and we were ready to go! The morning of the event, I felt sick and so nervous. What had I let myself in for?

Well, another successful achievement and challenge completed - that's what I'd let myself in for!

I have completed other challenges since and I can honestly say, I look back at each individual challenge and feel quite emotional. Each one made me face different fears, fears that I never thought that I would overcome. But I did, and I did so with friends and people who believed that I had it in me.

Facebook memories and Time hop are wonderful things because not only do they remind me of all the wonderful things that have happened over the years, they also remind me of the person I was prior to 2011. I've learned so many lessons along my journey, one of them being – you get one chance at this life so make the most of it. Look after yourself, mind and body and this will then give you the opportunity to take in all the lovely things that nature has to offer you. Oh, and if possible, do it with friends and loved ones.

Some reflections from my training diary… Go on…Make those memories!

Day after Three Peaks Challenge

How do I feel today – in a word, AMAZING!! I have just completed a challenge of a lifetime, something I never dreamed I would be able to do or want to! 3 Peaks done! What a feeling. I am surprising myself all the time and achieving things that I never thought I could!

Why did I do it? Well, reason 1 is that on the 1ˢᵗ June some of the V1ntage gang walked up Ben Nevis. Initially I thought that they must be mad. I asked myself, why? See, I have never been a big walker, so I just didn't get it. Not to mention I am scared of heights so the thought of going up a mountain over 4000ft high did nothing for me, apart from fill me with fear!

There was a lot of excitement on the lead up to the walk, I still didn't get it but on the day of the walk I felt excited for the gang. I followed their progress on Facebook and twitter, the more I read/saw the more it affected me. I wanted to be with them – not because I felt I was missing something but because I could feel something in my stomach, their sense of achievement and support for one another. It was amazing, they were amazing! My decision was made, I was signing up for the 3 peaks challenge. Me! I texted Gareth the day after the walk to let him know and to tell him how I had been inspired by everyone and what they had achieved. That was it; I was committed (or needed to be)!

Reason 2 – I wanted to do it for me, simple as. The 3 peaks have been discussed on and off since I started at my gym and I had always steered clear of the conversations because I thought it was something that I would never be able to do. Well, I know differently now. There was only me stopping me from doing anything. My Dad always said 'there's no such word as can't' and he was right. I can! That's what I say now.

A lot of effort and hard work went into the preparation for the 3 peaks. First big challenge for me came when I was on holiday and making sure that I didn't lose focus. Bournemouth and Weymouth are beautiful locations to take a walk, so it wasn't a problem to do a few miles a day. They are both quite hilly, especially Bournemouth. To get down to the beach, there is quite a steep cliff and in previous years I have been very lazy and used the lift up and down the cliff. Not this year, I walked up and down at least twice a day as well as going for a long sight-seeing walk.

Next was the practice walk from Anglezarke near Bolton, Spitlers Edge. I was obviously getting serious about these 'walks' because I bought some proper walking trainers!

It was a beautiful day and the group was in good spirits. The walk itself wasn't too difficult even though I had worried myself yet again because I wasn't very experienced. That doesn't mean I didn't ache the next day because I did – my legs didn't like the walk leader very much! I felt great after the walk and couldn't believe how much I had enjoyed it. The walking bug was getting a grip of me. There were so many positives for me – getting fitter, stronger, meeting new people and the scenery! I couldn't believe I had missed out on all that for so many years.

Now it was time for the serious stuff, Helvellyn – clue's in the name! On the run up to the day, I was getting quite excited even though I had seen some very scary pictures on the internet. I did a little bit of reading up to prepare myself. It did help in that I had an idea of what to expect, forget that the pictures scared the living daylights out of me.

I drove to the meeting point in the Lakes with my two friends Theaks and Betty. The mood was good in the car and we were all set for the big 'walk' – then I looked ahead. What on earth was I doing? I didn't like heights! Why was I doing this?

Panic started to set in and I was getting jelly legs. Not a good start! Theaks put a stop to me moaning and showing my fear, a few stern words from her and I shut up.

We started the walk from Wythburn Church, a beautiful location on a beautiful day. Theaks and I set off first because the rest of the group were waiting on late comers. When we set off, the start of the walk seemed quite steep and I began to worry about what I had let myself in for. I was *knackered after 10 minutes and began to stress over my ability to complete my three peaks challenge?! That fear didn't last that long. The higher we got, the more amazing I felt. I loved it and was surprised that I wasn't scared – well, not really.*

It is hard to describe how I felt at which point because I don't know the names of the different sections of the mountain. What I do know is different emotions took over at different times. There was doubt, there was confidence (at this point I was being shouted at, to watch my heart rate because I was racing off), fear and then there was astonishment. I just could not believe the views. Why had I not done this before? It really was something special.

As we neared the summit, I started to get a little emotional. I had actually done it, the top of the mountain in sight. What I didn't expect was being invited over to the cliff edge to look at striding Edge. Had I not told people that I was scared of heights? Oh yes, I had! Gareth has a way of making people do things and shockingly, I did go over to the edge - with more than a little encouragement. In my head I had convinced myself that I am never going to attempt Striding Edge but in my heart, I knew I would.

Just looking at it filled me with fear, but I knew it was a challenge that I wanted to take on one day.

Once I reached the summit with other members of the group, I had to stop myself crying because I didn't want to look silly. A lot of the group were experienced walkers and I didn't think that they would understand. This was a big thing for me, getting to the top of a mountain when in the past I would get in the car to go to the corner shop. My whole mind-set had changed. The scariest bit of this challenge for me was the descent. I remember reaching the top and feeling elated then I looked down and my first thought was – oh shit! I did it though and that is what matters. I overcame a fear (sort of) and successfully completed the challenge. Now I wanted to do another one and it's a good job really because Gareth already had the next one planned – Snowdon!

Snowdon was planned for the end of August, so I got some walks in of my own around Bolton and carried on with my training sessions in the studio.

I decided that I didn't want to set off to Snowdon first thing in the morning and booked in a B&B the night before so that I could rest properly. My bag was packed with energy gels, food, drink, plasters etc and I was raring to go. Snowdon was a longer walk and higher than Helvellyn, but the aim was to complete it in less than 4 hours. The thought filled me with dread, but I knew we would do it.

Not sure how I knew, but Gareth has a way of making you believe that it will happen, and it generally does. My confidence was higher at the start of the walk, but I wasn't complacent. I knew it would be tough and it was, but nothing worth doing is ever easy. All the same emotions came into play and there was still the same fear factor, but it didn't create any barriers for me. I was getting up and down that mountain and it was as simple as that. One of the things that I enjoyed most on these walks was the encouragement and support that the group gave each other. Without this I am not sure I would have done it.

The next challenge was the Bolton Cycle Sportive that I foolishly told Gareth about. I say foolishly because there were two options for this event – 35 miles or 60 miles and it doesn't take a genius to work out which option Gareth chose. Something seriously wrong with that man's thinking!!

Not taking on the challenge isn't an option, so I resigned myself to the fact that I would be doing 60 miles and started to enrol other V1ntage members to do the same. I felt good about doing this challenge not just because I enjoy cycling (even though I have only done it a couple of times as an adult) but because on the booking system it was named after me – how cool! After looking at the route for both the 60 and 35-mile routes, it was decided (thankfully) that the less experienced cyclists would do the shorter route – phew!

The event started early on a Sunday morning and one of the gym instructors was leading the

35 milers. Gareth was taking on the 60-mile route with the more experienced riders. My route was tough and at times I didn't think I would complete it. Either that or I would be walking the route! There were some tough hill climbs but with the group encouraging one another, we completed the challenge and I didn't walk once!

These challenges have changed my mindset, these group sessions are what I love, bring it on!

Gareth

I asked Kelly Burke to write a chapter for us because I know for sure that her 'journey' started with the same doubts and reluctance that may affect some of the people that might buy this book.

Kelly is proof that a spark of inspiration can lead to some amazing results and experiences.

I was with her for the entire weekend of her three peaks challenge and whilst there were a few times during that weekend that she drove me just a bit nuts, her efforts made me so proud.

Our aim was to complete the challenge in 24 hours and whilst I'd tried to get them to aim under 22 hours as we started in Fort William that Saturday afternoon, I sensed Kelly for one would be beyond delighted with just a sub 24 finish and, of course, that has eluded many people in the past.

Some creative accounting gets used on The Three Peaks by some folk, but for me, you set foot on the Ben Nevis path at say 4pm and therefore you must be back at your car with three summits bagged by 3:59pm the next day, there's no other way.

Kelly did this with Andrew, Jackie and me, and whilst it's by no means unique nowadays, it did, most importantly, give Kel' two things, wonderful memories and a kick start into a new mindset.

Why wouldn't you?

111

Louise Marie Mort & Russell Clifford Brooks

When I was really young I never understood why my dad used to go out running in the middle of winter in the dark. Me and my sister loved our roller skates, bikes and generally the outdoors, but Dad would run at all hours in the snow, rain, and cold, and sometimes carrying weights in his hands up and down Sharples Ave. I wondered, what's all that about. We thought he was mad. Until we went with him - and there it all began.

My relationship with running, fitness, netball and basically anything I could get my hands on physical activity wise began. Throughout school and college, it was my only real focus. I'm not sure why, I wasn't academic, but doing stuff that was hard made me feel good and that's all I knew!

Don't get me wrong, there have been times in my life where I have left this alone for some time, drank way too much Strongbow and enjoyed life to the max. But, somehow, in the tiny back space of my mind always regretting not having those feelings you get when you're on the moors up Winter Hill running through the trails just before it goes dark or in the early morning. Then, I have turned back to hard physical activity and this, in the last 10 years, has been one of the main focuses of my world. These feelings found me in a way. Always encouraged by my friends and family, in my thirties I have hit the training hard and achieved some goals I would have never dreamed of whilst rolling about on my roller skates as a young girl, or at 5am in the morning stumbling home from the 10th night out in a row in Magaluf!

The running was always the key for me (and my partner Russ who you'll hear about later), and it will always be the one I turn back to. You just need a pair of trainers, that's it, and a little bit of 'I will mentality' to get yourself out of that door, and those feelings come back, the accomplishment and satisfaction you get after a run, the "clear your head factor", is a perfect tonic for any problem, helps you think clearly. After a run, "problem solved" (well not quite, but it certainly puts problems and life into perspective I often find).

After doing spin classes at the gym for many years combined with my running, I started to "up" the training and could feel myself getting fitter, combining the two in 1 training session before work was making clear differences to my fitness levels and I started to look for other goals with which to challenge myself.

It started with my local Park Run and that wonderful concept I would recommend to everyone as a brilliant way to get into fitness.

That simple 5km run had me hooked. I had to beat my time each week and I loved the competition. Then came 10km races and then the half marathons. And then I was starting to think about triathlons. Not sure why, it just seemed like the next step. I didn't know much about them, but soon learned from mags and on line the basics – well you think you know…

My sister and I had, for a few years, had a "day out" watching the ironman and I had often declared, pint of cider in one hand, chesterfield cigarette in the other, "Sis, I will do that one day", but had never really thought

I would be fit enough, the distances involved made my stomach turn. But I did begin to wonder.

Not long after, I booked my first sprint triathlon with 2 days' notice, it was all very haphazard - one lunchtime on the internet feeling the need to do something new, I saw it, it was full, so I emailed them with a sob story, booked it, and turned up! The day prior to the triathlon I had to "check" I could do 20 lengths. I could always swim but am just about average and always will be. That doesn't bother me. I now look at this as the thing I must do at the beginning of a triathlon. 20 lengths done coughing and spluttering my way through the salt water pool at Nantwich, I jumped on my "mountain bike" and was off – this wasn't at all like a spin class, much harder on the Cheshire lanes with the thickness of the tyres on my several years old, never used, Halford's mountain bike. Perhaps I should have thought this through. Onto the 5km run and then I was done, a lot of 'should haves', but lessons learned. Some people train for years for their first triathlon, but there's nothing like jumping in at the deep end – literally, if you fancy it, go for it and learn as you go!

I met Russ not long after this and, having done his first Ironman, he was training for more. A similar background to me, we knew each other from our Bolton Wanderers spectating days. Russ had pumped the weights in his muscle-bound mans' gym in Farnworth forever, and had turned to running and Park Run like me in addition to his other training.

His story inspired me even more to believe in myself and I booked, and completed, my first Ironman in 2015. I never actually 100% believed I could do it, but I trained hard, I didn't use any fancy plans or weighed my food or let it completely take over my life, but I did what I felt I needed to do to get me through to the finish line. Each week I would focus on what I thought I needed to, trying to get the balance right between the 3 disciplines. Included in this I did lots of competitive events to keep the motivation going and to keep the drive alive, I treated this as part of my training. I set myself a goal of 14 hours. And, with 2 minibuses of friends and family following me round all day, it was an emotional and successful day and an absolute delight to cross the finish line. It was the same for Russ on his first ironman the previous year, he had dozens of family and friends supporting him along the way, which really does keep you going when you absolutely need it.

After the ironman, I wanted more. I felt it was crucial to keep going and set myself new goals.

I didn't want to be a "1 hit wonder" and I also knew I could do more.

Russ had a goal of 10 ironmen, of which we have now done 2 in France and 1 in the Pyrenees, the Altriman, at the time of writing, our latest ironman conquest which is voted one of the hardest in the world. And, believe me, I doubt there are many harder. We started in the water in the dark and eventually finished after midnight 19 hours 10 mins of blood, sweat and quite a few tears. This was Russ' 10th, and supposedly last, ironman, but I doubt this will be the case, with next year's events looming, I think we both know deep down there will be at least 1 or 2 more.

We have also both developed a passion for Trail Ultra Running. This has seen us do many mega challenging running events in some stunning places as close to home as the west Pennine moors, the cairngorms in Scotland and as far away as the Angkor Wat Trail – Cambodia. You can't really train for an ultra, we never knew this, we have just gained knowledge from others, because you can't exactly go out on a training run and do 55 miles, you just need a level of fitness that will get you through, the belief that you will do it and the endurance to carry on going.

These events are challenging, and you must pace yourself, switch off, enjoy the scenery, and get yourself to that finish line. Battling with your own self (as well as the pain in your body) is probably one of most difficult factors. You can be on your own for many hours with your own thoughts and can find yourself going a little insane at times. But the miles do pass by – eventually, you might go through your whole life story, and thinking about loved ones and memories you have but the miles drop away.

The key is to keep it positive and visualise that finish line, and it will come… eventually.

Most recently we took on the 'ring of fire' event which is a 135-mile trail run around the coastal path of Anglesey. Over 3 days there are time restrictions on each day and with a high dropout rate almost 1 in 2. There was a chance one of us wasn't going to succeed, but if you knew me or Russ you would know that neither of us would let it defeat us. Without discussion prior to the race, we knew neither of us would be that "one" in two, though we both secretly had our doubts, our worries and fears. Jesus – if one of us hadn't have done it, life would have been quite difficult for the next year! And so it didn't defeat us , we both completed the Ring of Fire 2017, we both learned a few lessons about looking after your feet and blisters, eating enough and the navigations skills required, nonetheless we both crossed the finish line in 1 piece (just about) to the sound of Johnny Cash (that song will never have the same meaning again as it was used at the start, the finish, and each morning to wake you up at 4.45am it will always bring back so many memories for us).

Suffice it to say, Russ and I love a challenge, and we are both quite competitive in events and with each other. There's nothing like having a training partner who is also your partner in life and love too. To reminisce on past events where we often have different stories to tell, people we met and mimic each other on our success and who did better – which is hand on heart usually Russ (though it's out of pity on my part more than anything, of course!).

To achieve something together makes it so much more worthwhile. There are rarely any "niggles", only during training over direction or distance, where we are both always adamant we are right. One memory that stands out is on a recent recce run of the Bob Graham Mountain Challenge Leg 1 which, due to poor navigational skills (note to always plan these things), an 11-mile trail run took us over 8 hours and through numerous rivers thigh deep, over fences, walls, barbed wire, one way then back the other, lost in the middle of nowhere with not a soul in sight. 24 miles later we arrive at our start point. It's safe to say we nearly killed each other on numerous occasions that day!

But we laugh about it now.

We spur each other on in everything we do and find new and exciting challenges to keep ourselves focussed. We like to see different places and compete in random events with often very few competitors. Our travels in the last couple of years have taken us to Morocco, Holland, France, Cambodia, Spain, Scotland, Wales, Ireland, and many a trip to the Lake District, one of our favourite haunts, and beyond.

All these events have brought so many emotions, memories and experiences

I'm not very good at constellations I barely know the difference between a Mars and a Galaxy, but I know what heaven is, it's over Holyhead Mountain at the finish line of the Ring of Fire after 135 miles running the coastline of Anglesey, or in Les Angles in France as we came down the mountain on our second lap and approached the finish line in darkness. You can barely describe the feelings and emotions you go through on these events, and to go through them together and experience the same things makes it twice as enjoyable. These are all sleeping memories now, but they will always be there. They are ours, we have been there and done that!

We have banked some fantastic times and memories that will be with us forever. We are so lucky to have done the things we have done together. 10 years ago, neither of us would have believed that we could achieve what we have done. But we have, and we will continue to seek out new opportunities and challenges together and hopefully encourage and inspire many others along the way

We are no experts, but we love to have a laugh about everything we do and have lots of fun along the way. We will never be scientific and understand the rules of rest, recovery and nutrition. We are just normal people who love what we do. We love a beer and to watch football like everyone else, we thrive from encouraging others and giving them our knowledge based on what we have experienced in this mad journey of ours.

We have met so many amazing people and new friends along the way who have touched our lives in different ways. Many will be friends for life. We love to support others around us and encourage and help them any way we can to reach their goals

The training and events we do are just a way of life to us now, one that we would never change.

We are definitely not pros, but what we have got is the drive and determination to believe we can do things and we both constantly tell people we really do believe that anyone can do anything. You just have to believe in yourself and that's more than half the job done.

Gareth

Louise and Russ are by some distance the maddest competitors of all my friends, and, later on in this book, you're going to read another of their massive successes, but for now I want you to focus a bit on this, they are both just ordinary bods like you and me

I mean it, they got started with easy stuff, but before they did, that easy stuff had eluded them!

They just decided to start something different and I know for sure that neither of them knew where it would lead. Nowadays what they have is a shared passion for the same type of exercise. A shared passion for travelling to unusual places and hey, these two do stuff on a budget too, then compete together.

They just found a great way that they really enjoy, to keep fit. Running mainly, I think they will agree, the swimming and cycling though is still at a very good level, but they enjoy best their running.

And remember what Louise says 'After you've bought the running shoes, there's not much else you've got to buy'

Park Run, is everywhere, why not check out where your nearest one is if you're struggling to find a way into running. The social atmosphere at Park Run is amazing, trust me, go see.

Andrew Stewart - My Fitness Journey

I was never a sporty kid at school. My parents were not
interested at all in sport. At school, I ended up stuck in
the second row or on the wing. My parents despaired as
I developed an interest in (watching) football and my
passion for Newcastle United. Growing up in arctic
Northumberland, playing cricket was pure torture, as I
literally froze.

Roll onto my first term at Christ's College, Cambridge,
and I thought I would have a go at rowing, which was
the first sport at which I had both success and
dedication. I was so unfit when I started out – I can
remember the pain of my first run along the riverbank.
Nonetheless, I developed fitness, strength and an
appetite and worked my way up from Novice VIII to 3rd
VIII and then 4 terms in the College 1st VIII. I carried on
rowing when I started working in Southampton and had
two successful summers rowing with BTC
(Southampton) ARC, winning two Hants and Dorset
Championships and one South Coast Championship.

That was when the fitness and exercise stopped. I
became an unfit and moderately overweight
thirtysomething, especially during our five years living in
America.

Approaching my fortieth birthday in 2004, I started to
become aware of my own mortality and health,
especially as I saw my father deteriorate with
Parkinson's Disease. Exercise wouldn't have helped
Dad with his condition, but I started to think much more
about my own health and how I could approach the
second half of my life in the best possible form. I entered

the Great North Run, my first half marathon, and set off on a training programme of regular running that got me from Newcastle to South Shields in 2:13.

As I started a new job in 2007, I was on the road much more, and started to take my running shoes on trips to keep fit and cope with the hotel food. I ran another Great North Run in 2008 (2:02). The running was fun, and it was also great to raise money for charity.

I kept running once or twice a week. In 2011, I entered my first Great Manchester Run (10km in 57'04"). Having run around 200km in both 2010 and 2011, I set myself a goal to double that distance in 2012 - I split the goal into running 10km/week, with a grand total of 558km for the year, knocking 5 ½ minutes off my Great Manchester Run time.

My fitness journey really took off in 2013. Around New Year, I was having coffee with my mentor and friend, Dave Evans. He asked me if I would consider entering the Manchester 100 (mile) cycling event in September 2013. My first thought was hell no! I couldn't possibly cycle that far and, anyway, I didn't have a bike. When I had an email in April about the Cycle to Work scheme, though, I took action and got a bike. I went to Halfords with Callum, my son. I was thinking of a mountain bike, but he persuaded me to get a road bike.

I fell in love with cycling!

I loved weekend rides with Callum, and often with his friend Jack and his father, Ian. We all decided to enter the Manchester 100! As a practice, on Yorkshire Day, 2013, the four of us cycled 122km from Bury to Thirsk. At the time, it was a monumental goal – and so satisfying to arrive at my Mother's house. We all completed the Manchester 100 a month later.

Exercise became an extremely important part of my life. Not only was I active – strength training, running and cycling – but I started to study nutrition. I made some major changes to my diet, doing my best to minimize my consumption of processed foods and sugar. I read a lot about how the body processes sugar (Dr Robert Lustig) and some of the emerging literature which debunked the previous government advice that we should have low-fat, high-carbohydrate diets.

I had been attracted to the idea of running a marathon for several years, but had never had the courage to enter one, fearing the pain and the commitment. So, at Christmas 2013, I took the plunge and entered the next year's Greater Manchester Marathon – it was the year of my fiftieth birthday, after all! Before doing so, I researched what it would take and developed a training plan, with the help of the excellent book "You Can Go the Distance" by Bruce van Horn. He split the training into three runs per week – a distance run at the weekend; a tempo run, and an interval run. The distance runs were hard at first. I had run two half-marathons (21.1km) – as soon as I did my first 25km training run, I had problems with my feet (blisters and almost losing a big toenail). Once I sorted the right pair of shoes, I was OK. My typical distance run was Bury to Manchester Victoria, 30 - 32km with a nice stretch through Heaton Park.

Race Day was fantastic. I had raised £800 in sponsorship for Parkinson's UK. My goal was to complete in under 4 hours. I set off behind the pace setter for 3:45. The first half was great. As soon as I hit 32km (the furthest I had done in training), I was up against my mental wall. At that stage, running past Carrington, my legs were in pieces. It hurt to run, and it hurt to walk. Those 5km were the toughest of the day. I got to about 37km and realized I was only 5km from the finish and I chanted to myself "I'm going to finish a marathon" and suddenly everything was easy again! I finished in 4:08

Dave Evans called me again one day, a month or two later, and asked if I would like to join a cycling trip to the French Alps the next year. My answer this time was HELL YES! At the end of May 2015, I ended up in a car driving to the Alps with three Ironman trainees (Dave Evans, Gareth Price and Rhauri Mundy). We stayed in Le Bourg d'Oisans, at the foot of the legendary Alpe d'Huez. Nothing that I had read or watched prepared me for the unrelenting brutality of cycling up alpine cols (nor the exhilaration of lengthy, outrageously fast descents). In England, it's almost impossible to find a climb that is longer than 5km. In the Alps, you can find yourself grinding up a 20km climb that takes 2 hours or more. Memories of that year: the amazing 1000m descent into Séchilienne; getting to the summit of Alpe d'Huez and the brutal 40km drag up to the Col de la Croix de Fer. At the top, it was hailing and snowing, and I did not have my winter kit with me. My hands were so cold, that it was almost impossible to change gears until we had dropped 500m altitude to some warmer roads. The lower part of the descent to the Barage du Verney was as good as any descent I had ever done – smooth roads with sweet, gentle, bends.

Earlier in 2014/15, I had done two consecutive 60 Day Challenges at V1ntage fitness studio. The challenges involved six workouts per week (mainly Insanity) and an intense focus on nutrition. I got down to 80kg and the fittest I have ever been.

Gareth, Dave, Chris Twist and I went back to Bourg d'Oisans in 2016. The highlight was getting to the top of the Col du Galibier at 2640m. The descent, once past Col de Lautaret, is such a wonderful experience, except for the terrifying journey through a dark, rutted tunnel at La Grave!

After we were back, Dave called me again (there's a clear theme here… and I should have said no). We discussed entering La Marmotte, but it was full, so, instead, we came up with the idea of entering the Tour du Mont Blanc. Described as the world's toughest one-day cycle race, it takes riders 330km around Mont Blanc, from France to Switzerland to Italy and back into France. And it has 8000m of climbing! The challenge was accepted.

Like the marathon, I realized that I would need to do some special training. The goal captivated and frightened me. I enrolled in a training course run by A1 Coaching in Dublin (www.a1members.com) and I dutifully went through the base, build and peak training for 7 or 8 months, through the winter and into the spring. I was on really good form as we went to France for our June training camp. We chose a different base and did some different Cols in 2017 – Col de la Madeleine; Col du Glandon and Col de la Croix de Fer (from the north side) and then the Daddy of them all – La Marmotte, leaving out Alpe d'Huez.

Tour du Mont Blanc took place in mid-July. Four of us took part – Gareth, Dave, my son Callum and myself. We arrived on Thursday and spent Friday preparing, relaxing and registering.

3:30am the alarm goes. Up and force down coffee, porridge and bread. Check bottles, lights, spare kit and get dressed.

4:45am on the start line with Dave. 500 plus cyclists in the dark, with much nervous energy.

5:00am we are off. Amazing to see a snake of red bike lights heading off down the mountain towards Megève.

At about 5:45, we have some daylight and some of the high peaks are illuminated. On we head towards St Gervais and Chamonix. The first big climb up the Col des Montets, then a high-speed descent across the border and a brutal 12km ascent up to Champex. We were feeling good -- we had made the first cut-off with plenty of time to spare. We had probably the best experience of the day – an extremely fast descent on long, straight, roads with amazing views over Martigny.

Once past Martigny, reality struck as we started the 25km climb up to Col du Grand St Bernard. Grind. Relentless. Grind. Not as steep as Champex (until the last few km). Rest in the wind at the top (just into Italy), then the descent into the Aosta valley. This descent was not as enjoyable, due to the strong, dangerous and gusty wind.

Callum and I were ahead of Dave and Gareth. We heard about their progress from our support team, Debbie.

126

Dave overheated and was violently sick on his way up Gd. St Bernard. Callum was suffering.

We made it down to the bottom, and the furnace that is Aosta. Callum decided to drop out at La Salle. I was in two minds as to what to do. It was 4pm and we had an 8pm cut off at Bourg St Maurice. At that point, it was 52km to the top of Col du Petit St Bernard, plus probably another 30km descent. I didn't think I had a chance of completing that distance in time.

In the end, the broom wagon passed me after another 15km and I decided to quit. I could have gone on, but I would have been on my own and unsafe. In the end, I felt so proud that we had put our bodies into the arena and given it a go. Disappointed we could not finish, but proud.

What's Next?

Since returning from Mont Blanc, I have really enjoyed doing some unstructured bike rides with no training purpose. A few friends have suggested I enter Ironman 2018 – I can't say I will never do Ironman, but it is not on my agenda for 2018. Maybe 2024, as another epic challenge for a landmark birthday? I am going to enjoy the last months of summer on my bike and then keep myself fit through the winter, ready for the Alps (or Pyrenees) next year. A sportive or two, but nothing like Mont Blanc.

Twenty years ago, I was 91kg. I'm now 82kg and fitter than I have been since my University days. I feel great and intend to keep it that way.

Gareth

Andrew sat on a yoga ball in my studio in 2012. He wore chino slacks that sported a sharp vertical crease, a smart well-tailored jacket and an open collar shirt. A pair of light tan brogues, I was guessing Grensons or Jones, and the most outrageous pair of socks I've ever seen.

Truth is, I can't remember exactly, but you've got the picture now.

On a positive note, the socks matched. 5 years later, knowing him well, I'd say those socks said everything about him, crazy design, but perfectly matched.

In July 2017, after cycling for 12 hours, 150 miles and 7500 metres of vertical ascending, having had just a shower, this lad jumped in a car and drove two hours at midnight to rescue me from my own Mont Blanc challenge.

If it were possible to put in a bottle the message we are trying to get across in this book, Andrew personifies it and if we could wring him out, that's would be where the essence of success could be found.

He always does what he says. Always!

He's tasted the success his hard work has brought about and, clearly, he's not about to go back to his old ways. He's Made things happen for himself, he's found that which enables his Exercise to be fun, his Nutrition is balanced, and he enjoys the good stuff in moderation. He's put the U in MENU and he's on track for a healthy and longer life!

He also reminded me recently about a speech made by Teddy Roosevelt which we both think is extremely apt:

THE MAN IN THE ARENA

Excerpt from the speech "Citizenship in a Republic" delivered at the Sorbonne, in Paris, France on 23 April, 1910.

'It is not the critic who counts; not the man who points out how the strong man stumbles, or where the doer of deeds could have done them better. The credit belongs to the man who is actually in the arena, whose face is marred by dust and sweat and blood; who strives valiantly; who errs, who comes short again and again, because there is no effort without error and shortcoming; but who does actually strive to do the deeds; who knows great enthusiasms, the great devotions; who spends himself in a worthy cause; who at the best knows in the end the triumph of high achievement, and who at the worst, if he fails, at least fails while daring greatly, so that his place shall never be with those cold and timid souls who neither know victory nor defeat'

David Evans

ALTITUDE 2017 - Climbing Mount Evans

The first encounter of the massive mountain.

My first visit to Mount Evans was by car. We had a Ford Expedition. A huge thing, designed to conquer most terrain and it made the Range Rover I drive in Britain look small. An American muscle four-by-four. We drove up the most impressive highway the I-70 known as the highest 3-lane road in the world, stopped at Idaho Springs and made our way up towards a little place called Echo Falls.

We drove the first 4 miles to a visitor centre where we parked up and walked to the viewing deck, Goliath's ledge. The road was perilous, there were huge sections where the side of the road had no barrier, just a vertical drop, direct to the valley or cliff edge, whatever was below. At first, when you get out of the car at 12,000 feet with no time to acclimatise, it is a very strange experience, where you feel almost drunk and nauseous. We had decided to walk the 2 miles relatively sensibly, given how weird we felt, taking just a small part of the walk at a time. Initially 0.3 of a mile and stop. It soon became 0.1. The reason for explaining this is that the altitude had a huge impact on what we thought was going to be possible.

The density of air at sea level around the world on average is 750 Tor (which defines the amount of Oxygen in the air). Denver Colorado is a mile above sea level and sits around 620 Tor at any given time. The summit of Mount Evans is 460 tors.

Driving the road, although scary and challenging, made an impression on me. It gave me the desire to want to come back and cycle it.

Taking on the Challenge of Mount Evans

The ride later came to take on more purpose when I was invited to speak at a conference in Denver with a hugely successful business called Payroll vault. The theme was Altitude. It got me thinking, let's take the ride on, with the conference theme in mind.

We arrived in Denver on Sunday, flying in from a few days in Orlando. Mid-afternoon, the CEO of Payroll Vault, Sean and I, went to the local bike shop where I had arranged to hire a lovely carbon American Trek road bike. Step one - planning.

Planning for the RIDE - planning for your challenge

In business or pleasure, challenge or leisure, planning is critical. Thanks to my experiences riding in the heart of the Tour De France in the Alps around the Bourg D'Oisans area and the wonderful slopes of Alp D'Huez, I had been given the opportunity to learn the importance of planning. For the Mount Evans challenge, I had decided that I needed several things in order to complete it.

- One: Tools and kit, to be safe on the ride

- Two: Items from my road bike back home, saddle, lights, helmet

- Three: Weather-proof clothes for varying temperatures. Warm weather and cold

- Four: Fuel

- Five: Enough water for a longer ride (at least twice the distance)

- Six: Local knowledge and riding expert knowledge

Items gathered, prepared, packed - Step One done

Step Two: Decide your outcome up-front.

In business and in challenges like this you also have to decide up-front your level of commitment to the challenge. Something we sometimes forget to do in business is to stop, take stock of things and think about multiple outcomes.

- What is the outcome I want from this challenge? Result?

- Are there key situations to think through? Success / Challenge / Failure / Set-backs

- Who else is able to assist with the outcomes?

- What is my level of commitment along the way?

- Answer the questions that say…'What will I do if X?Y?Z?

This was a critical phase for me. I was climbing the mountain to conquer it, to have the thrill of being able to say, I rode to the top of America's highest paved road and succeeded. I also wanted to capture the learning that takes place when your mind forces you to make choices and decisions under extreme pressure. In this case, the literal physical pressure, caused by lack of oxygen.

Step Three: Set the date, mark the calendar, GO!

Once you have gone through the steps and preparation, once you have the focus needed to take on the challenge, it's time to press the 'GO' button and start. For me, it was the 21st of August 2017. It was the morning of the famous Eclipse, it was time to ride at Altitude and see what happened next.

Start Point Set: Idaho Springs - Target: Mount Evans Summit

The Ride itself.

One of the suggestions presented to me around the early effects of the Altitude came in two different forms. The first was that somewhere between 11,500 feet and 13,000 feet was where I would find it really challenging. Confirmed by cycle bloggers who talk about the last couple of miles.

The second was that the first hour, was the critical part.

I unloaded the bike, went through the last couple of pieces of preparation, fuel, water, sun cream, seat height, shoes, glasses, sweat cap, and we were off.

The first mile was an interesting affair, the journey up the road was 15 miles to Echo Falls, where there is a little Lake and turn to the foot of the official road up the Mountain. This first stage is far enough, it is climbing, it comes with its own challenges. The cycle shop had suggested starting from the turn point. For me, that did not make sense. The thought was that the first part would allow me time to adjust to the oxygen depletion. After all, one day being in the area was not enough to adapt to the air. That mile number 1 had lots of things going on. My heart rate was going faster than normal, the initial gradient allowed me to vary between 10mph and 13mph which was confusing. Eventually, as the gradient changes, you find yourself slowing right down on the corners with climbs in them and the speed drops to more like 7mph and 8mph and then to an eventual 6mph.

Both parts of the climb have mile markers to let you know how many miles you have climbed. I have grown to like these from riding in France, where every Col has climb markers measured in km which also tell you the average gradient of the road. No gradient guide here, just the miles - I figured this was better than nothing. Mile 1 done and soon a relatively fast five miles, in fact the fastest of the day - 34 minutes. I was settled into the initial altitude. The physical feeling is a blend of nerves and sensory override, the closest thing that captures this is the butterfly feeling you can get in your stomach when you are nervous. The road rolled around the lower mountain through forests and long ranges. It varied in style with some classic bends that go back on one another and eventually, a little while later, I arrived at the most serene little lake again called Echo Falls. By now I had done 14.5 miles, I could see the turning to Mount Evans and was ready to meet with the same road I had seen on the car journey a year before. Throughout the first part of the ride, Debbie supported me in a small SUV, providing pre-filled bottles and support. This was critical to reduce any stopping, so that I could keep my body in a balanced state.

The foot of Mount Evans

Vast mountain ranges tend to start on top of another mountain. Mount Evans is exactly this. Taking the turn, I began the lonely climb up the mountain. The signs reset to zero and I set off in pursuit of the first mile.

Those first few miles in fact to mile 5 were most peculiar. It was around the time of the solar eclipse. The temperature on the mountain dropped by 15 degrees Fahrenheit and I added additional clothes at the bottom. The lower part of the mountain had been in the high seventies. The road here was narrower. The conditions for cars were treacherous, the terrain was more rugged, and the quality of the road began to gradually deteriorate. Soon enough, I arrived at the viewing deck, next to the visitor centre and, feeling quite pleased, I pulled into the car park, switched more water with the support car and immediately continued.

Leaving the centre, the scenery changed significantly, the terrain at the side of the road lost its trees, the mountain became more barren, the road more isolated and the first of the long curving visible stretches lay in wait. In total, there were at least five of these prior to getting to the next landmark, the lake at the foot of the last climb; Mount Evans Lake, five miles from the summit. These long lonely stretches were surreal, they were beautiful to look at, you could look off either side of the road and see right into Denver Colorado over multiple other valleys and roads. Each one forced you to slow down, manage your breathing carefully and take it one step at a time. The altitude was climbing with every pass.

Eventually I got to the lake, having passed a herd of Elk, and I saw Debbie in the support car for the last time. This was the point where you take on the last five miles. The road from here is ridiculous and narrow, it made sense to do it alone. Debbie went back to the visitor centre and I carried on. The approach to the final five miles is somewhat cruel, you get a half mile descent, where the bike picks up from 7mph to 21mph. What is cruel as you go around the left corner at the lake, is you know on the way back this was one of two small sections, fatigued and tired you would simply have to deal with. I turned the corner and began the longest 5 miles I have ridden. While mathematically the distance is the same as any other five miles I have cycled, this was the hardest, without a doubt. Reading the blogs about it on the way out to the USA, I would read comments like 'It is a fair comparison to Alp d'Huez in France and like, many cycle fans, I would scoff at the idea. Yet it is reasonable and truthful to say and I admit that it is. The effect of the oxygen as each mile goes by, messes with your physiology, interferes with your thinking and, when you put these two things together, it quite simply messes with your mind.

By now, the markers were at 9 miles, 10 miles, 11 miles, going up and up. Being in double digits was fantastic. The mind wandered to getting back to the support car some 9 miles to the visitor centre and through lots of thoughts and feelings running through my mind. The longest mile took place between 11 and 12, it was a point where I passed a cyclist who shouted not far now, he was one of 3 I saw all morning. I was riding through the part of the day where the Altitude was reaching its max one bend at a time. I remember feeling fatigued and heavy, an effect of the air. The strange thing was, I did not once feel challenged on muscle power or fitness. Just heavy and experiencing the need to drink continually. When I hit mile 12 I was so pleased, knowing that there was only 3.2km to go. When we train in the Alps I particularly love the markers when they get under 10km and then under 5km. I imagined them to be present to help me break it down into smaller mind steps. Mile 12-13 was hard. I was at my worst from this point to the actual summit 14.5 miles up the road from Echo Falls. I stopped at a half mile point, to fuel, drink and eat. Taking 40 seconds to do it. The experience of stopping was weird, as your heart rate falls you feel weird, almost dizzy, 40 seconds was long enough to settle and go again. The strangest thing in the world is knowing that moving is easier than stopping. Your brain thinks this through and finds it confusing. The advice at the beginning was spot on, the altitude at its worst is found in the last 2 miles. I don't know what point I passed the 14,000 feet mark, all I do know is I felt it.

It was during this last 1.5 miles to the top that I became concerned about the descent. The thought in my head was as follows - 'What is the effect this weird physical feeling is going to have on me when I turn to descend this mountain? Will I be safe? Will I be able to concentrate?'

The final mile.

In business, we meet so many people who settle for mediocre or quit too soon. You can sometimes be so close to success or achieving a goal, yet you can become too weighed down or frustrated by the amount of commitment you are having to give that stopping can seem like a sensible choice. This was a critical point for me. I felt ill, I felt weird, each corner was still going up, the road was narrow and rugged and awful. Apart from one moment of total serenity, the road was a beast. In the final mile I was forced to do one thing. Break it into three parts, a third and a third and a third. Sometimes the win is achieved in smaller steps, with patience, determination and grit.

Applying my plan, I climbed and hit the 14-mile marker, turned the next couple of corners and took in the golf ball igloo shaped building and hit the summit. Riding alone and without any haste, I turned around and started descending. The fear of not being sharp enough, or safe on the descent soon left my mind. Earlier, I mentioned how bad the road quality was. It really is bad. The mountain bikes you can hire with super suspension would find some of the holes in the road tough to withstand let alone a road bike. Nonetheless, it was time to go. With juddering shoulders, I focussed the core and the upper body and bounced my way back down. It was brilliant to see the miles and speed sky rocket and the time per five miles decrease back to normal cycling speeds.

The road in the distance

There is a moment in the last five miles where you climb up and around a series of bends to go over a false summit, as you climb, you get to see this road in the distance miles away across two vast mountain plains that look like a fake picture. The road seems fuzzy and unreal, yet it was clearly there, it left me feeling philosophical and wondering where it went, who rode it, why was it there. It is also a great visual memory of leadership and how we can sometimes wonder where the road ahead is. The secret, of course, is to keep moving forward in whatever endeavour you have chosen long enough until you are able to reach the point at which you can discover the answers for yourself. The answer, after all, is almost always nearer than we might think.

The descent was glorious - one of the wonderful experiences of road cycling when you climb is the joy of descending and, once I got to the Echo Falls main road, I was able to enjoy some safe and fast speeds to the bottom. I particularly enjoyed hitting a top speed on a hire bike of 51mph and the incredible buzz doing a 5-mile stint in 8 minutes.

My Mount Evans climb had purpose to it and during it I was able to learn many things. The thing that stood out to me though was the following reflection. Decide your outcome up-front.

Setting your all-in commitment up front is a vital step when taking on a challenge. Knowing the answer in advance when a situation unfolds is critical. For me, it is vital. When the last two miles presented some colossal breathing and body issues, my choice before the ride to continue, break it down and use my intelligence and experience, predetermined that, unless I was literally sick, I would be continuing.

The challenge of Altitude takes real guts, in business and in sport. What is your altitude ambition, and have you developed the L in altitude enough? The 'L' being Leadership - the self-Leadership to commit yourself to your goal and your purpose.

I remember Dave saying to me in 2014 that his black touring bicycle, that had set him back a modest £750, was the best value spend of his life, even then, and having influenced him a little in that purchase, it made me smile.

Today, he's midway through ordering his dream bike build, a sexy black Pinarello F10, as ridden by Team Sky, who speed past him daily on his rides in Majorca. They do have one thing in common, though, it's their training ground.

Like the velodrome sessions I take part in, cycling is one of the few sports that allow us wannabies to 'compete' on the exact same terrain as the best in the world.

What chance you footballers can rock up at Old Trafford, Anfield or Wembley or your own favourite football ground and have a game of five a side on the pitch, none!

This book isn't about getting anyone to do anything they don't want to do. Quite the opposite…but I for one am throwing cycling in the mix for you. It can be as high in intensity as any form of exercise, it will burn calories, get you fit and fluctuate your metabolism as needed.

It's easy on your joints and, contrary to popular belief (in the context of spinning in particular) is not bad for your knees…Just sayin'…

Tim Huxtable

Can I? Can't I? Will I? Why wouldn't I? What if I fail? Is failing an option?

The same questions I would always ask myself when taking on a challenge.

Then I remember the five 'P's; Prior Preparation Prevents Poor Performance.

Fail to prepare therefore, prepare to fail.

So, the simple answer is to train and dedicate the time. Put in the effort and reap the reward, in all walks of life. Whether it be cycling, swimming, walking, cross country, Couch to 5k.

Two examples I would like to share with you. First, the Coast to Coast to Coast Cycling Challenge in July 2008. A 230-mile, 24-hour, cycle challenge starting in Sunderland on the east coast, reaching Whitehaven on the west before heading back east to Sunderland. The challenge was simple; start at 6am and return by 6am the following day.

There were four of us taking on this challenge, but I knew I wasn't fully prepared. I hadn't trained as much as I should have. Work and family life all play a part, but doesn't everyone have this excuse?

The rest of the team were fit as they were training for Ironman, so I had the extra pressure that I would slow them down. Would they wait? I'm not good enough… I'll just go halfway I said to myself. That way I would have challenged myself, earned the Coast to Coast medal and let the stronger riders complete the overall challenge.

However, teamwork is exactly that. Mind over matter, pull together, anything is possible. My mind-set, *our* mindset, was to focus only on the next 15 miles, at which our support driver would be waiting for us.

When I reached that goal, only then focus on the next 15 miles and so on and so on until the adrenaline kicked in and the finish line was in sight. And what a feeling that was! Hard to put into words. That feeling exceeded all expectations. Emotionally overwhelming and unbelievably satisfying and great to share it with my team.

Could I do it? Yes!

On my own? No!

Never underestimate the importance of teamwork and community spirit and positive thinking to reach your goal.

Walking is another interest of mine, especially mountain walking. The freedom of being away from everyday life for the hours while up on the mountain is, in my opinion, priceless. If you get the weather, the scenery can be stunning.

The concept is the same – set a challenge, a goal, a target that tests the limits. Give yourself a realistic timeframe so that there is enough time to prepare. Set the plan, stick to the plan and enjoy!

The second challenge I want to share with you is the national 3 Peaks challenge which I've enjoyed taking part in on a number of occasions where the purpose is to climb Ben Nevis, Scafell Pike and Snowdon within 24 hours. Each time I have taken park I have beaten the 24 hours - delight!

Why? Because the team I trained with all shared the same goal. To succeed!

Yes, I can train and make myself mentally and physically prepared, but what about my team mates? How do they feel? Are they ready? The team is only as good as the weakest link.

Help each other - positive thinking.

Anything is possible with time invested to prepare. I always doubt that I am not good enough, but on many occasions, I have surprised myself. Perhaps I can do even tougher stuff if I put my mind to it.

And that's the point. Yes, you can!

Gareth

No, really, listen to him!

Yes. YOU. Can!

Find a way, but start off looking for that 'way' by knowing that you can, like Tim and me, enjoy exercise so much. Exercise which fits into your life rather than forcing your schedule and diary to accommodate exercise.

Make it irresistible in your life!

Tim is a busy lad, he's got a family who he is devoted to and a demanding and responsible job. He enjoys an extended family and a large circle of friends, and has a busier social life than most, but, he stills find time to keep in great shape.

For now, I want to take you and him (when he reads this) back to our Coast to Coast challenge and please bear in mind this is my recollection of events and may vary from his.

It's about midnight on the return leg of our coast to coast to coast, 24 hour ride, we are heading east along the A66 towards Scotch Corner. We are at around 2000 feet above sea level, and despite the time of year, mid summer, it's only a few degrees above zero.

Remote and desolate!

We are riding in line, our bicycle lights glowing in the dark and we see a car ahead in the layby, it's our support driver Bill, the red lights at the back of his Ford Mondeo are again, a welcome sight to us all, we are all suffering with aches and pain, about 180 miles under our belts in this epic 24 hour ride.

'I've had enough guys' says Tim as he unclips his shoes from his pedals and climbs wearily off his bike, lifts his back straight one more time after our latest 15 mile stretch of unrelenting hill.

We look at each other, Lucy, Neil and me, a little shocked I can tell you. It came from nowhere, but unlike the Kilimanjaro moment and a few times in my life where others have hit their wall before me, a contrivance of little things changed his mind.

I deployed a little persuasion his way and asked him to join me on the beach at Sunderland as we dipped our toes, ceremoniously in the North Sea, I wanted to share that golden moment with my buddy!

Our driver Bill has got his mileages 'wrong' and even said he'd worked it out on the GPS, urging Tim to see off these last 34 miles!

Long story that, but let's just say it was a blessing and a curse.

Tim finished the C2C2C challenge with me in under 24 hours, it was a stand out achievement in my life and I know in his too!

Make a stand out memory in your life, find that thing that will do that for you and help you to be fitter.

Louise Mort & Russell Brooks

Kodaikanal Mountain Ultra 27th January 2018

When people mention the word "India" the first thing that pops into most people's minds is curries, poppadums, temples, the Taj Mahal, Gandhi, dehli belly and cricket!

I doubt the majority of everyday people would imagine that they would one day be running through the mountains of India as part of a 130km Ultra race through the night. However, that's a decision me and Russ made (possibly after a few too many glasses of wine) on a cold winter's night in not so sunny Bolton. It was a choice between that and another icy cold run up to Winter Hill, it was a no brainer for me! (with a cheeky holiday added on the end as our motivation for getting to the finish).

I had stumbled across the info for the 1st ever **Kodaikanal Hills Ultra 2018** whilst "browsing" the internet. Not sure how I actually found it if I am honest, but it popped onto my screen as if by magic and rattled about in my head for a few days – I definitely wanted to know more.

Russ and I had both been to India before, but we had never run this distance before, this certainly seemed like it could be an adventure and definitely a challenge. So, that was it, decision made. Just like the Beatles did in 1968, we planned our magical mystery tour of India (minus the Hashish, getting high and writing a hit album!).

I started to research were this place called "KodaiKanal" was, the logistics of how we would get there, the finer detail around the race etc. And of course we hatched a plan to have a holiday afterwards, my goal being us relaxing on a beach somewhere, after running 130km through the mountains. Language barrier always a blocker, I emailed people who I could find had an involvement in the race to find out more. It's not easy sometimes, getting people to reply to your emails, and understanding the info they are giving you.

The key thing I needed to know was, where in this vast country were we going and how would we get there?

I also needed to know a little about the race, the terrain, any time restraints and if there were direction markers – visions in my head of being lost in the middle of India being quite an important factor in our safety on the trip.

Getting little bits of info at a time, the trip began to fall into place. Not the easiest place in the world to get to, though. We booked our flights into Chennai and then started to add in the finer detail of the trip.

Transport in terms of buses, trains and flights in India is pretty cheap and easy to sort, but the country is absolutely huge so what on a map appears to be not far at all, can be hundreds of kilometeres, and they don't have the M6 or St Peters Way (Bolton's A666 urban motoway) knocking about. Some of the roads are rough and ready, and you always have the odd cow or monkey to negotiate along the way, which adds to the fun of the trip.

I worked out we had to get into Kodaikanal a couple of days before the race to acclimatise. The race was due to start at 3am in the morning to allow certain parts of the trail to be covered in daylight that would have been dangerous in the dark (always a confidence booster being told that, NOT!).

I booked an internal flight to a place called Madurai where we could then get a 3 hour bus ride or taxi up into the mountains to KodaiKanal, in the state of Tamil Nadu.

Prep for the race – many people ask us how do you train for an ultra, or an event such as this?

Many experts would probably argue with me with many scientific facts, however we don't feel you can train fully for an ultra, you can't just bob out on a Saturday morning for a quick 50 miler. You have to think about how this effects your body and your recovery too. The key for us is about maintaining your fitness, and time on your feet.

So, in the couple of months preparation we did have, we did some hill walking, a difficult trail marathon, and, prior to that, a 40 mile trail. Longer spinning classes also helped, and adding a run immediately afterwards, again time on your feet and keeping moving, getting your body used to working for longer and harder.

So, after a flight to Chennai via Frankfurt, a short flight to Madurai, and a taxi ride with tea and monkey viewing stops (several), which we didn't ask for - the driver just kept stopping and ushering us out of the car. We drove through the mountains up to the hill station town of Kodaikanal. At over 2000m the town is literally in the middle of the mountains with stunning views in every direction.

In the usual crazy Indian way there little tuk tuks, buses, cars, dogs, cows everywhere and constant noise. Bizarrely, due to its location, it's a busy town with a bustling market, shops, and apparently well-established boarding school, which is one of the best in India.

The school, it turns out is the registration, start and finish point for the race. We were the only Europeans that had entered the race, it was a truly international affair.

After acclimatising for a couple of days, which involved us celebrating Russ' birthday in a local bar with a few beers and dark rums, not the ideal prep for a race but our training was done now, we had bigger fish to fry than worrying what effect a few beers may have on our quest.

Our attention turned to the race and the small question of, how do you get your head around running 130km?

Answer is simple, you don't!

The main thing is, with any event whether it be 5km, 130km or a triathlon or ironman, you have to believe you are going to complete it, and want to do it, and see yourself at that finish line, what's in your head is the only thing that will get you through. And, if you have the determination and the will to get yourself there, that's half of the battle.

Of course, being in the middle of India, a couple of other minor considerations and concerns we were hoping to overcome. Not least, the fact that we had only been in India for 3 days, the time difference (plus 5.5 hours) and start time of the run and ensuring we had enough rest beforehand.

We spent quite a lot of time walking around KodaiKanal but tried to ensure we had 2 good sleeps before the start.

Food – Having a staple diet of "curry" before the race wasn't the best idea, but it's really difficult to find the usual foods you might have at home, and the traditional "masala dosa" for breakfast probably wasn't the energy food we were looking for.

We managed to get omelettes and toast at our hotel and I managed to find a restaurant that did Pizza and Pasta, which was our chosen meal the night before the race.

During the race, nutrition would be a huge challenge, there were due to be a number of aid stations but the description of "Salt, sweet, energy and water" left their actual content to our imagination.

Climate – The temperature in KodaiKanal was varied, at night it was surprisingly cool, as low as 5 degrees, and, during the day when the sun was up, it was between 25-30 degrees.

We had to be prepared for this, starting the run layered up with additional clothes in our packs for when the sunrose, and again for when it went dark again. In addition to this, we needed a litre of water at all times, and usual bits such as blister plasters, spare socks, Vaseline and, last but by no means least, toilet roll!

We always carried a compass, but neither of us are navigational experts, Russ is often likened to a naughty

Labrador, and never listens to what usually is the correct direction (a one and only subject we often disagree on). So, we ditched the compass and a few other 'un-needed' items to keep the packs as light as possible.

We had both learnt a really important lesson in a previous race in Anglesey that I mentioned in my previous chapter, called the Ring of Fire. During that 3 day event, we had both suffered badly with our feet. One of the key and most important things to take care of on these longer events is your feet, because you really do need them!

If you start to get blisters, you have to act quickly, you wouldn't believe something so small could have such an impact on you and cause so much pain, but, believe me, it does, and it hurts! We both knew this and with the heat, we planned to change socks and Vaseline our feet throughout the race to prevent the inevitable from happening again.

Race day!

After a few hours drifting in and out of sleep running random scenarios through our heads, we walked over to the race start for the briefing. It was quiet, it was pitch black and we both felt apprehensive about what lay ahead for the next potentially 28 hours (the max allowed for the event).

Runners for both the 130km and 80km events were due to start at the same time, and we drew quite a bit of attention to ourselves being the only Europeans, the only female being me from what I could see, my blond hair, and Russ's not so quiet voice!

Lots of selfies with random Indian people took over the pre-race nerves, and a random Bollywood style warm up with music, which I watched with disbelief!

My warm up will be the first 10 miles, I thought to myself.

A minimal race briefing followed which sticks in my mind, but mainly it consisted of…

"beware of the bison – these are big bulls"

"the first part and final part of the race is a hunting ground for them"

"if you see one, or hear what you think could be one, turn off your head torch"

"hide till they go, or walk past very quietly"

"don't look them in the eye"

"don't run alone, especially you females"

"follow route signs at all times"

Well – that's the most interesting and motivating pre-race briefing I have ever heard, I thought. In fact, it couldn't be any worse! On the bonus side, no mention of tigers or snakes!

Within minutes we were lining up at the start line and before I knew it we were off.

Whilst thinking about the race the last couple of days, I had thought to myself, "well we can't go any higher so the start of the race must be downhill" I had convinced myself of this, and thought it would be a good warm up, but clearly I was wrong. They had somehow managed to find a hidden mountain and at least the first hour was spent running upwards, in the pitch black, wondering what the hell I was doing.

The Beatles track "Help" sprung to mind. One of the distractions was the amazing skyline, with a clear sky – possibly because we were nearly in space! The stars looked amazing, I had never seen so many clusters of stars and it almost felt like I could touch them, I couldn't stop looking at them, I will attribute blame to the stars for my snail impression detailed below.

I must admit I felt awful the first couple of hours. Russ had a spring in his step and I could tell I was frustrating him going at a slower pace and he was annoying me making a point of giving me the Paddington Bear Stare and looking at me in disgust at each bend we hit.

Hitting the second aid station, I told him to go on ahead, which had always been the plan of attack. I needed to get my head around the task ahead, without feeling the guilt for not being Mo Farah for the first few miles.

My dad's words rang in my head "don't worry about what anyone else is doing, just worry about yourself".

Anyway, on the clock ticked.

The miles (or kilometres as they talk about everywhere else in the world) began to tick away and time went on.

On these long runs as we both could tell you, your thoughts run away with you and you can more or less think your whole life through, but the one thing you simply have to do is keep it positive.

Going for a big run can often be a great problem solver, help you think straight and see everything in your life very clearly.

Both Russ and I have family and loved ones we like to think about. Russ has children and grandkids who are very dear to him and who he dedicates all his events to. I have my friends, parents, sister and niece, who are often at the forefront of my mind.

My thoughts often turn to my Grandad who was a war hero, and I often think about what he did for our country and motivate myself by comparing the mere run or event that I am doing to what he went through in the war, and pray for him to look out for me. (I didn't include the bison in my prayers to him, though he definitely wouldn't have approved).

As each aid station passed by, I checked Russ' progress and at only 13 minutes behind him at about 30 miles I had a little smirk on my face as the thought crossed my mind that I could catch him, and he may have started too fast (I secretly hoped). I would have loved to see his face as I caught him, he would never live it down, that little smirk kept me going for some miles.

We are quite a competitive couple, but mostly I do come off second best, but, if I don't, he certainly knows about it!

The feed stations were interesting

- Slices of cucumber or tomato with a pile of salt or the option of all 3 on a slice of bread
- Lemon or lime slices with the pile of salt

- Some sort of peanut cluster type thing
- Bananas
- Water

Given the unusual choices, I opted for the slices of tomato and cucumber dipped in the pile of salt – and swished down with a mouthful of water, I convinced myself this would be the best option. Having not felt great, I didn't want to eat anything substantial at this stage and thought that salt over sugary would be best for me given the temperatures expected during the day.

I kept thinking "just need a tequila with that", looking at the salt and lemon, but perhaps it's good they didn't have a clue what I was on about. I had my own electrolytes which I added to water and ensured I kept hydrated throughout this was key and I stuck to it.

It became light around 6.30am and I had started to feel really good. Looking back, I think when it came light, and the sun was shining through the mountains and I could see the most amazing stunning scenery I can't even begin to describe, I couldn't help but feel good. I was glad I was there, and was thankful for having the opportunity to see some remote parts of the world most people will never see.

I had no reason not to feel good!

The cliffs and mountains were broken up with forest trails into valleys where little villages still slept and would later begin their day to day activities, filling up their water from the well, doing the washing in the river, burning things. Running through one village it was call for prayer as people made their way to the temple at dawn, I smiled and waved as I ran through.

Each village had children in abundance, who were absolutely fascinated at our passing through their village running alongside us smiling, asking our names, and high fiving us!

I even gave away my "emergency Haribo" for some of them to share as they ran with me barefoot through a village. I wanted to give them a treat or something, water or a plaster was all I had otherwise!

I hope I don't regret this, I thought, as they happily shared them out.

Russ, still ahead, I later found out was running with a guy we met the previous day at registration, from Chennai, a runner from the local running group, who we called Mo Farah. We were both running strong and Russ felt particularly good, he was picking of a few of the other runners as the miles ticked away.

I had caught up to 2 runners who I continued to run with for the next few hours. Language was always a barrier, but just having someone at the side of you gives you the comfort you aren't lost and helps keep your pace.

We chatted a little, the younger guy from Chennai had run the distance before, and was hoping to finish in a decent time, the other guy was from North India, and in the Indian army, he didn't carry a pack which astounded me in the heat, he said as part of his training in the army they go for 2 days with no food or drink, he was happy to get water at the aid stations and took only a banana with him each time!

The thing that astounded me most was that that he had literally sat on a train for 3 days to get to the race start, 3 days on a train, no changes, no get offs, just 3 whole days on a train! As you can imagine, this fascinated me and he must have thought I was insane as I kept questioning him about it , although I don't think he had a clue what I was on about, he kept saying something to the other guy either to clarify what I was saying or probably to question my sanity!

I haven't mentioned much about how we felt during the race and broken it down mile by mile because I think it's important in any endurance event to keep your mind occupied with positive thoughts, your surroundings and keeping things real by breaking down the tiniest of hills into tree by tree and the bits of race that are the toughest into ever smaller sections.

It's safe to say, however, that the whole of the race was mountainous, at altitude. It was difficult to breath at times and, with 10,500ft or so of climbing, it didn't really bare thinking about. But when you ran down the valleys into the nice little villages with all the nice people waving and high fiving you, in the back of your mind you knew that a ginormous hill was about to appear just around the corner and try and destroy you.

Being the tough old cookies we are, we weren't going to let a few mountains get in our way (there's a song in their somewhere).

Along the way, I often occupy myself with songs, how many Prince songs can I remember, relevant songs to what I am doing ie. Ain't no mountain high enough, or reverting back to the Beatles again "hard day's night" and other random stuff to pass the time.

I think you find yourself slowly going a little mad with your own thoughts on these endurance events, perhaps a little delirious in your own thoughts, but amusing to look back on at the end.

Russ didn't know where I was on the race, although I knew he was asking about me at the aid stations, and I was checking his times, he was gaining on me, whether him getting faster or me slower he was now around 45 minutes in front of me.

Funny, I thought he would have got lost by now!

Being a little bit older than I, I started thinking perhaps he's been here before, maybe with the Beatles!

So, with darkness approaching again me and the Indian army guy lost track of the young runner, he dropped behind and we caught Mo Farah who told us Russ was running well, but Mo was starting to struggle.

We ran together for the next couple of hours and shared food and drinks as we miscalculated the next aid station, the Indian army guy was struggling and rested a couple of times.

At the 58 mile feed station I still felt pretty good – changing back into my night gear, "my anti bison protecting long sleeve top I thought". This feed station has masal Dosa, rice and chapatti which was definitely at the bottom of my requirements list at this stage in the game.

Knowing that Russ wasn't hanging about either, I decided to leave the station on my own, whilst I still felt good and get as far as I could with the daylight I had left.

Other than the last 10km, the last section of the race was more or less all uphill. Both Russ and I had very similar experiences on the final mountains.

This involved me shedding a couple of tears as dark drew in and I started to tire, but I knew I could get to the end, I was just willing my legs to keep moving.

Picking off one tree in the distance to use as a goalpost, then picking off another. Ignoring the random noises in the trees and darkness, I chose to leave my headtorch off as much as I could and use the moonlight for sight, though this didn't stop me from seeing some Green eyes looking at me from the trees.

I glanced sideways, then glanced again to confirm they were actual Green eyes, and then kept my head forward didn't breath or make a sound and sort of ran tip-toed for the next half mile with a limping whimpering style.

I didn't look back. We reached a point where a family of bison had been spotted. Each runner then got an escort from the race organisers for about a mile or so with a jeep on their left with 4 people positioned on the back. There was also a person either side walking. At this point, I had the definite sensation of running, but, with hindsight, it was clearly not very fast, as these people were just walking alongside me

I was now feeling very anxious about getting to that finish line - it really couldn't come soon enough!

My legs had taken all they can. The organisers were now saying it was safe for me to go alone, and I had 15km left, mostly downhill; it felt like nothing. They said another mile or so and I would see some street lights which was the start of the town of Kodaikanal.

I made them promise that they weren't lying to me, and I remember keep saying to each of them "promise me it's 15km and no more"? I am not sure why I was convinced they were lying to me it must have sounded like I was starting to lose my mind.

I underestimated how much my legs had taken a battering and it now appeared that running downhill was much harder than uphill – in my head I had planned to fly down that last few kilometres, but there certainly wasn't a flight left in these legs nor Russ', a shuffly type jog thing was adapted – ministry of silly runs I thought to myself.

What they failed to tell Russ or I was that there would be 3 thousand stray dogs roaming the streets, coming up to you having a sniff, running round you in circles, standing barking at you, or just watching as you ran by, or, better still, running alongside you.

As if the Green eyes, potential bison, random crunches and cracks in the woods, weren't bad enough, now another potential hazard. I am not surprised we knocked up 86 miles, dodging cows, dogs, and bison. And that's not to mention if there were any snakes and tigers, murderers and kidnappers!

Approaching the town, a feeling of elation creeps into me, yet still a few miles to go. Having reflected on this afterwards, we both thought we were nearer to the finish than we were, and there were a couple of extra twists just to finish us off and then we found ourselves approaching the lake by the school to finish!

I became a little dis-orientated and as it was just gone midnight, there weren't many people about, plenty of dogs though, I decide a quick phone call to Russ (who usually ignores me) but assures me I was on the right path – I had an accompanying dog with me as I attempted a sprint finish across the finish line and I was done.

Russ finished in second place and me in third!

Delighted with having accomplished this massive task, our holiday was in sight.

Now just shivering we had no hot water for a shower (typical India), so we found as many dry clothes as we could and huddled up in bed together shivering away with thoughts of what we had done going through our minds.

A few hours later and we were back on our feet. We didn't sleep well. We had made the wise decision to get moving the next day (not) and get a 3 hour bus ride (flat tyre = 5 hours) followed by the overnight train down to Kerala for our holiday.

The race hadn't quite sunk in and we had hardly spoke about it as we stumbled up the street to the liquor store, bought a Kingfisher beer and sat on the pavement waiting for the bus.

We could hardly believe what we had done, and later in the holiday on the beach and at various points, different aspects of it would come back to us and though we didn't run together, our experiences and thoughts and feelings about the whole thing were similar and chatting through different sights and scenarios helped you realise just what we had achieved.

Sleeping Memories now, they are there at the back of our brains, stored away, never ever to be forgotten.

The race was all for charity so although we each achieved a podium position, we didn't receive a prize but that's where the memories are. The funding from the race will go to building sanitation for one of the schools we ran by, which beats any prize for us.

People think we must be mad and say they don't know how we do it.

But, as I have said, you just keep moving, one foot in front of the other. As with anything, the hardest part is getting off that couch and out of that door. Then you can do anything you want, anywhere you want. Who cares what other people think. It's your life, don't let another year pass you by, if its park run or marathon des sables who cares, it's what you want - go and do it!

Gareth

The most recent story in this book is Louise and Russell's India epic event. It would be easy for you to have enjoyed the read, but maybe to dismiss their stories as far too hard to even contemplate. But, before you do that, I'd like to tell you about a relaxed chat I had with Russ after India

As Louise explained in her first chapter, Russ started his running at the local 5k (3.5 mile) Park Run. He used to lift weights and wanted to increase his overall fitness.

We were chatting about events we'd taken part in that had 'beaten us'. For me, my Tour de Mont Blanc and Russ explained how his first mountain marathon went - he barely managed half of it and had to beg a local pub to call him a taxi and give him a glass of tap water to help him recover.

He told me how he drove past that pub for months on his way to work and it drove him to enter, train harder for, and to complete that same race the following year.

The difference may just be the desire to improve. Sure, Russ and Louise push each other hard and they take on some massive challenges, but they both started out small and look where it took them. Did they know where it would take them when they both got started, no!

They are the perfect demonstration of the Goethe and Roosevelt theories if you ask me.

What separates you from them or anyone in this book? Trust me - nothing does. Why not see what you're made

of, like all of us here, we started and built the parachute
on the way down. Avago!

Ironman UK: My Story Gareth Price

It would be easy to start my Ironman journal on race day, Sunday morning, 1st August 2010, my first attempt at this mega challenge, my toughest at that point in my life and, at exactly 2:40am as I lay awake with just over half hour to getting up time, wondering for the millionth time, would I be able to manage this mammoth task, wondering, had I just bitten off more than I could chew this time round, all the training was done, all my dear friends and loved ones had done their part to assure me I was ready, nothing had been left to chance, I'd done the hard yards, I'd really done the build-up stuff, 100%, completely!

And yet, why the doubt, yes, and the nerves? There's no complacency in this boy, no way, but why so very nervous, when I'd done everything I could to make myself ready? So many maybes, so many possible problems, not least my injuries and knee problems, no doubt about one thing, joint pain in my knees later in the day, but, amazingly, astonishingly, that one thing I expected and knew would happen, didn't!

Nobody had received more support than I had. The people close to me had proved the absolute value and need for everything that true friends bring to such a challenge and, for this competitor, they were such an essential factor in the preparation and, of course, the event itself.

Thank you everyone, I kept thinking!

I agree with Tim, Team is crucial, and the Team don't have to be competing with you either.

165

And, amongst those friends, my financial sponsors for my charity - such generosity, and, in case we forget, the money we were raising is so vitally important to help the local hospice do its thing, I was doing ironman, me, just having a fun day out, compared to the people at the hospice, who, sadly, may not even have the chance to take a walk, may not be able to plan, even to go on holiday, hey, Ironman, aint nothing man!

Game on!

Soon enough, the alarm for 3:20 sounded. I was out the bed, not so much like a coiled spring, more like a vintage car being cranked for the first time in years, but, within minutes, I'm feeling just about as good as I ever can at that time in the morning! Not a morning trainer me, never have been, but the training sessions I'd done had helped me be in a good place on this, the most important, day of the Ironman journey.

After a shower, a bowl of porridge, easily the biggest I'd ever eaten, was seen off in quick style, three bananas and a protein shake. Probably enough I thought, yep, my tummy was telling me I'd had enough, another success, getting all that down, when I'm not even keen on eating until after that first cup of filter coffee and maybe checking a few emails. Today, though, isn't any normal day.

My friend Tim is alongside me as we hear the doorbell go, Zoe is here to take us to transition one at Pennington Flash near Leigh. With her is one of the other four David Lloyd members taking part, Gary Davies and, at 4:15am, we are headed for the start.

166

The roads are quiet, but certainly not deserted, as we make rapid progress and arrive just as the queues begin to form, we parked carefully (rather too carefully by the Lady from the Rotary who I hoped would get more efficient as the morning wore on).

We chatted together, pensive, nervous, as we walked toward the bright lights, music and sounds coming from the main transition area. 1500 expensive bikes, all racked immaculately behind fenced barriers, I knew just how much time and money had gone into assembling all of that, it was quite a floodlit sight as we gazed across in the semi-dark.

Tim took a few pictures and even that served to crank up the nerves even more, butterflies in my stomach the size of eagles, bumping around inside me, but hey, this is what being alive is all about.

5am passed by quietly, the 6am starting gun was getting closer and closer, Gary and I made our way to check in, Zoe and Tim, giving us such a fabulous send off, the cool morning was still and dry, someone had smiled on me this day, calm water was mine, thank goodness for that, thank YOU to my guardian angel!

I smiled inside and out!!

As we entered the secure area, we were asked to get our legs and arms marked up with our race numbers. Marian who I'd recently met on a spin course, had been in touch to say she was on race number duty today, but she was nowhere to be seen. I'd looked forward to seeing her before we started, but much as I looked everywhere for her, in the 12 or so queues waiting to be done, there was no sign, we chose a queue and waited, moving slowly forward.

I looked left and saw Dave another of the David Lloyd entrants from Bolton, we checked with each other how we were? All ready!

The guy at the front of our queue, was just about to turn to leave and there I see Marian kneeling down, I'm next, yay!! Hugs and smiles, ace!

All marked up and ready to change into my wet suit. The atmosphere is now as close to electric as I can imagine. How can I explain how I felt? Well, I don't have the words, to be honest. Into the wet suit, which, I have to say, made the swim tolerable for me, it may be compulsory Ironman attire, but it's been a huge positive for me and helped me to deal with my nemesis discipline, even if I do look like a complete knob in it!

Hat and goggles in hand, I pack up my white bag of belongings which will be at the finish later and hand the bag to an official outside the transition tent, so well organised, seriously excellent!

There is a large gathering of competitors at the exit gate now. We are being readied for the walk down to the water's edge, deep breaths to calm the torrid feeling in my tummy, oh boy, this is it! Soon, I can prove to myself whether I can do this 2.4 mile swim in less than 2 hours 20 minutes or not, and for those that don't know, that is slow, I am, a slow swimmer, I HATE swimming!

Past hundreds of spectators now, all clapping. It's an exciting feeling, I have never experienced anything like this before. Even the London Marathon start, doesn't come close. I'm in a different league now, albeit at the foot of this league table. I'm in there with the best triathletes in the world today; this is awesome!

Ray McGloin, another of the 'Bolton Lloydies' taking part, appears. He's done Ironman twice before, his words of advice from days before, come flooding through, "stay out the water 'till the last possible minute, which I tried to do, but as I was so close to the front, the press of bodies became almost impossible to resist.

Gareth, it's time now, get in and just do it!

We all moved into the water, across a mat, and then tentatively across slippy boulders under the water. Instantly, I was aware of the algae, in between my fingers and even a piece in my toes, yuk!

I'm in, and I gently make my way toward the start, which, I thought to myself, is about 200 metres or more away. I think, crikey, as if 2.4 miles isn't enough, cruel...! As 6am approached, it was so crowded, legs hitting against me, arms touching me, but, unlike most of them, I'd be at the back, clear water, to be able to swim this in my own time, just focus on getting to the end of this in less than 2 hours, god willing, please.

Guardian Angel, help me please!

The end buoy of the first straight seemed so very far away, and after several minutes, it seemed just as far away, I took one look at my heart rate monitor, 8 minutes gone, and I swear it looked even further away.

Now, not to make too much of a deal of that distant marker, and not to make too much of the pressure I was feeling about this swim, but I was in turmoil as I allowed myself to believe that marker was, thank goodness, getting closer, it just seemed like it had taken far too long to get there. My mind was so active and only about one thing, could I get out the water, and not be ejected from the race for taking too long? Yes, it was doing my head in!

Eventually, I got to the end marker and allowed myself a look at the monitor, I can't even remember what it said, and nor did I know if this was equal to 40% of lap one or maybe less, but it gave me a smile as I quickly calculated that I was ok, this was a good feeling, if short lived.

I carried on and started settling back into the negativity of earlier, and as I approached half way, I was being passed by the elites. Then, Paul, a swim coach from my gym, shot past me and called out 'Only one more lap Gareth!'

Strangely, I remembered he'd told me he was expecting to complete in 55 minutes, so as I awkwardly made me way round the half way buoy, I allowed myself a look at the watch. 52 minutes, I was delighted, and finally I could relax a bit, just get this swim out the way, get on my bike and then I could focus on getting under the 4:30pm cut off for completing the bike course.

The rest of the swim was a struggle; always is for me, but at least I was able to relax a little, I knew I was safe now and focused on going as quickly as I could, I thought maybe try and save a few minutes. Push, push, push, it seemed to be taking ages, but I knew my progress was good enough.

With maybe half a mile to go, I was joined by a safety canoe, and the close proximity of the boat was really bugging me, but the incessant cough I'd got in the last half hour from the weird water meant it was all I could do to breathe as I swam, so I just tolerated him, as the finish came closer and closer, and, closer.

Finally, those last few strokes, I tried to stand up, the shore crew urged me to swim a few more strokes and then, they had hold of me, I was out. My legs felt rubberier than the material my wetsuit was made of, but after just a few strides I was feeling stable and as the deafening cheers of the crowd, especially Zoe and Tim, rang in my ears, I felt my smile crack my face......... yes!!

It was done at last, on reflection this felt almost as good as finishing!

'Hey mate' says one of the crew '.... Your timing chip hasn't registered?!'

I didn't mind, that was their problem, not mine, Zoe and Tim came alongside me, pictures, video camera in my face, both urging me on, congratulating me, Zoe knew full well how pleased I'd be with 1 hour 52 - it was the best I could have imagined! Never swam more than 2 miles before, how utterly chuffed was I, again, I looked up to the sky and thanked that guardian angel, who'd delivered on the need for calm water, thank YOU!

Transition team were awesome, I was out of there in about 10 minutes, I collected my bike and ran to the start of the ride, Tim and Zoe hollering at me 'Go G, go!!!!'

I tried to make a slick start but succeeded in getting the crutch of my tri suit caught on the front of the saddle and did a comical 180-degree spin which gave everyone a huge laugh, not least me!

'Other way mate, it's the other way' shouted someone - too funny!

Away, on it now, this was G time, the bike section, 112 miles, my favourite part.

Towards Westhoughton, and then Chew Moor just a few miles from my home in Lostock, I saw a weight lifter from the gym, Jud McKnight, who'd waited for me with cheers and waves, then though my own village. My wife and some friends from club. It was raining slightly now, but more cheers and whooping. Come on G, game on, MY ride time, then Vicky cheering me near her home, we'd seen David her husband who was competing at body marking earlier, yay. Half an hour or more gone now, the effects of the swim starting to wear off, time for a Mars bar, yum!

Sam and Richard to the Beehive just a few minutes later, more cheers, wow!!!

Then Steve Horrocks out on his bike, one of our training gang, fab! He'd been the rabbit to my overweight greyhound during my training, an amazing cyclist the perfect build and very fast. The route took me about 15 miles, to the start of the loop track which had to be completed three times, just under 32 miles each, through Adlington to Rivington village and the big hill, Sheephouse Lane. The first time proved to be the hardest and, already, I was being lapped by elites on

their fabulous machines, such power, such speed, I
have to say, I was in awe!

So many people cheering, so much support, invaluable!

The hill was conquered and I settled in, completed the
first lap and enjoyed the second lap even more. More
friends and, despite the stiff breeze that was getting up,
I knew my guardian angel was smiling on me and after
the hill levelled above Belmont, the highest point on the
course, never was that presence felt more strongly than
as I approached halfway with the open fells ahead of
me, wowzah, what a brilliant feeling!

Emotions so high, I was feeling very confident now.

Lap 2 done, the elites now all into their runs, it was time
to have some fun, picking off one rider after another, up
Sheephouse for the last time, Rivington village, more
friends Lucy and Neil calling out to me and, minutes
later, halfway up the steep gradient, the screaming and
hollering 'Team G' egging me on. Tim, Zoe, Sue and
Sheree in the pink hospice T shirts, shouting for all they
were worth, what a fabulous buzz, five or six more riders
overtaken, I was finally eating into some of the minutes
lost on the swim.

Finally, the big hill at Sheephouse Lane for the third
time, done, I hooned down into Belmont village, left turn
there, stiff but easy incline out into the moors, and I felt
utterly amazing again, the open fells ahead of me again,
I was flying now!

I may have even stolen from the finish line moment up
there, I allowed myself to imagine I was going to be an
ironman that day, realisation at last!

I'd moved up several hundred places by the time I completed the ride. Into T2, at the school and changed for the run, I looked at my watch, for the hundredth time that day, I had seven hours to complete 26.2 miles of marathon, I was over the moon, I was safe now, just a case of grinding out the run, avoiding injury, seeing it through.

So many faces I knew, such amazing support. Nothing technical now, not like the swim, which was tough in so many ways, just a mind game that had to be won, me versus that marathon distance, into Bolton town centre to complete the first lap and the tantalising view of the finish just feet away, but for me, another 14 miles to go. I collected my second coloured band to prove that I'd done that part of the run, then, almost back to the start, only to run back, third bangle safely on my wrist, just 7 miles of the course to go, lots of time, now, could I get there, power walking, jogging slowly, could I get there in less than a total of 16 hours, knock an hour off my challenge, could I?

Mile after mile, slowly, they ticked away, mile markers very much in absence I'm afraid to say, disappointing after such an amazingly well organised event, but I really needed them, wanted them, so I could count down. Then I saw 23 miles for the second time, this time, it applied to me, this time, I knew beyond any doubt at all, I had all but done my first ironman, nearly there....

At 9:32pm, I managed to muster my legs and ran the last few yards, up to and then along the red carpet to a noisy, amazing welcome, all the gang cheering and jumping up and down, and those words from the MC

'Gareth Price, YOU are an Ironman!'

I crossed the line, despite how fatigued I was, despite
the intense pain in my legs, I could only feel delight!

It was utter delight.

Before I went to the guys for pictures and hugs and all
that went with completing the fabulous challenge, I took
a minute, to say hi to my Gampy. This time, unlike
Kilimanjaro, only smiles. I also said another silent thank
you to my Guardian Angel, whose services I think I'd
won with all my hard work, and, without whom, I would
not have finished.

No tears now, just pure and complete, total joy, an
experience I went on to enjoy again in 2014 and 2015,
when a team from V1ntage Studio successfully
completed the event (more on that from Jackie later in
the book).

Concluding my reflections here, then, my message to
you is a profoundly simple one, if I can complete three
Ironman triathlons, anyone can do whatever they set
their mind to.

Liz Price - Reflections on an End to End

First, let's get the rider out of the way (if you'll pardon
the pun). I can make no claim to physical prowess, skill
or aptitude. So, if you're looking for sporting inspiration,
motivation or similar …there's nothing here to see, I'm
afraid, and it might be best if you head straight along to
one of the other chapters in this book which might better
serve your needs. If, on the other hand, you're happy to
travel with me through my reflections on a very long
bicycle ride, then you will be more than welcome.

Stories of sporting 'daring do' usually involve references
to the better health to be acquired from the activity and
the lighter body weight and multifarious positive
personal and social outcomes that will inevitably follow
(and therein, of course, lies their inherent motivation),
but this chapter is slightly different. My reflections here
certainly focus on one long cycle ride, but I might as
easily have used, as my narrative hook, any of the
physical challenges I undertook as a younger, much
fitter, and certainly more physically 'well' person. My
reasons for writing it are by way of a reflection upon a
changing embodied identity and the ways in which
declining health and physical ability and illness can
fundamentally impact upon our sense of self creating, in
the process, a vicious circle of 'daren't' and 'can't'
mentality. My reasons for writing it are that I would like
to think it is written with a view to generating a little more
'can' and 'will', whatever physical circumstances you
(and I) may find ourselves in.

Lots of the chapters in this book start at a pivotal
moment in a story and, as narrative strategies and

techniques go, I think this works pretty well. So, here goes…

It is 5 AM in the morning and I wake up with something of a start. It's day four of a very long cycle ride that began at a foggy Lands' End and will, all things being well, finish, some 15 days later, at John O'Groats. I still have upwards of 900 miles to cycle, but the way I feel in the murky early morning light suggests that the end of day three may have been my final destination. Suffice it to say, I feel very unwell indeed and stagger backwards and forwards from the bathroom (the activities in which, I will spare you) not entirely in full consciousness. My fellow cyclists, all completely new friends three days earlier, are concerned, as are the organisers of the trip (I imagine they were anxious about any negative publicity… Someone corking on your well-planned holiday doesn't look too good in the brochures!). They all suggest that, at the very least, I should sit out the day's ride in the ever faithful, but universally feared, 'Van', which is destined to follow us the length of the UK.

This potential hiatus in my plans was completely unanticipated. I had not been demonstrably unwell in the lead up to the ride and had trained hard (but probably not really hard enough) for the rigours of riding over 1000 hilly miles. The ride was in memory of my mother who had died, 9 months earlier, from liver cancer which had gradually, but brutally, dissolved her strength, but not her spirit, and I was raising money for my local Hospice. I thus felt a good deal of responsibility to successfully complete the challenge - frankly, I would rather die there and then than set one cleated cycling shoe inside the 'Van'.

Breakfast is simply out of the question, but I managed to drape myself over my bike and begin a very slow and stately pedal across the Somerset levels, flanked by concerned looking fellow travellers. By late morning, however, I'm starting to feel a little better and, after a brief cafe stop, we point our bikes at the Cheddar Gorge. I'm so pleased that I decided to carry on, because, as we make headway into the day's ride, my physical state visibly improves and, by late evening, when the day's ride is done, I really am not feeling too bad. Had I known then what I know now, however, I would almost certainly not have been grinding my way slowly up the country. Rather, I would have been better advised to cycle, as swiftly as possible, to the nearest hospital. More of that later, though.

Day four slips easily into day 5, which is pretty much indistinguishable from day 6. Get up, shower, eat, ride, eat, ride, eat (a lot) sleep. The rhythm of days in the saddle is steady, predictable and, for the most part, profoundly pleasurable. The miles slide steadily (if slowly) under tyres warmed in the heat of long late June days, the landscapes are, by turns, brutally hilly and gently undulating (but never flat, as the ride's organiser has a very evident penchant for taking the 'scenic' route) and I am treated to vistas that I would, otherwise, never experience. Friendships form as challenges are faced and overcome in the pursuit of each person's goals and ambitions and life on the bike is simple, physically tough and deeply rewarding.

There is, thankfully, no more physical drama for a while, save for the aches and pains that are expected and even welcomed during such a long ride. A brief encounter with Wales soon gives way to England again and I find myself in familiar territory in Chorley, Lancashire, where my father and brother, David, meet me with smiles, encouragement and lots of cake (which I have discovered, thanks largely to cycling, I have an almost limitless love for). Reluctantly leaving them behind, we push on towards the border and the rigours of Scotland (though I'm sure that anyone who undertakes the ride south to north would agree that the hills of Devon and Cornwall are far more challenging than those north of the border) where the Rest and be Thankful Pass is waiting for us with the worst weather I have ever encountered on a bicycle.

Tossed by wind and torrential rain, we fight our way upwards. A stop at a small café that clings incongruously to a bend in the road is where Billy (a life hardened Glaswegian who eats hills for breakfast) decides enough is enough and he is literally poured (for that is the extent of the rain heaving ceaselessly down from a night-black sky) shaking and pale into the Van. Next, two young women are blown off their bikes as we descend towards Inveraray. They find themselves upside down in a culvert running alongside the road, at which point we are passed by a posse of motorcyclists who hoot and wave. I can't imagine they are enjoying the weather much better than we are. They look utterly drenched and our own group is becoming increasingly demoralised.

179

I am simultaneously afraid and exhilarated. Cold to the
bone and, like Billy, shaking uncontrollably, I am
becoming concerned that I will be the next person to be
swallowed up by the 'Van', but the rigours of the
weather present a challenge I feel impelled to
overcome. So, we continue down and down for what
seemed like hours. The decent is never ending. I
already knew that I had Reynaud's Syndrome at this
point, so the effects of the cold were, for me at least,
extremely challenging and I imagine I lost multiple digital
capillaries on that one descent alone!

We reach the foot of the pass and have ten miles to go
until we arrive at Inveraray. I am now certain I will not
make it, so we take shelter in the first habitation we
have seen for some hours, which just happens to be a
rather upmarket fish restaurant on the shores of Loch
Fyne, where I spend at least an hour warming my hands
under the hand dryer in the ladies' toilets. The staff are
more than tolerant of a small gaggle of very soggy (and
possibly rather smelly) cyclists rendered
incomprehensible by the cold. They ply us with hot soup
and crusty bread which, as it touches the sides, fends
off the incipient hypothermia just a little. The second and
third helpings certainly kick-start the process of thawing
out.

As we sit shivering and giggling at both our misfortune
and good luck, the motorcyclists who had passed us
earlier in the day reappear at the restaurant. They say
they were concerned about us when they passed us
earlier and that they came back to make sure we were
ok…I am almost tearful in the face of their gallantry, my
labile emotions not helped by the fact that I do not feel

too good and do not relish another ten miles in the saddle before reaching a soft bed and more cake and chocolate (the only things really guaranteed to restore a sense of equilibrium at this stage, I fear). Nonetheless, on we ride and, upon reaching the night's B&B at last, I spend the evening completely prostrate, wishing that it were possible to mainline Mars Bars. But, a warm shower and some much needed rest render me almost human again and ready for the next day's ride.

There is certainly something to be said for overcoming what appears to be insurmountable physical adversity, but, even though the next day's ride takes us through the most beautiful and remote Scottish scenery, I am anxious in case bad weather strikes again. It is an anxiety I carry for the rest of the ride. I think yesterday's drama has taken its toll and I am clearly at a low physical ebb. Again, though, a slow and steady pace and lots of scones at a lovely waterside café (in the middle of what seems like absolutely stunningly beautiful nowhere) helps the miles go by.

It is a day or so later that I again experience physical problems that seem out of proportion to the size of the actual physical effort I am expending (albeit recognising that cycling ones way up the country is a singular feat of physical endurance). We had stopped to eat at a very remote pub in the Highlands, but, despite not having eaten for hours (something of a miracle in itself), I had no appetite whatsoever. As my companions tucked into steaming food, sandwiches, cakes and all manner of other tempting energy replacers, I simply fell asleep, literally slumped on a bar stool with my head, still encased in my cycling helmet, on the table in front of me. I have a vague memory of being poked and shaken as fellow cyclists tried to wake me up, but it was extremely difficult to even open my eyes. I have never felt so utterly physically deplete and there was little to do but drink as much caffeine as possible and take on board much needed sugar. I'm sure that any nutritionist worth their salt would take issue with this approach but, in the absence of anything better, coffee and multiple Mars Bars really seemed the only way to go. This physical full-stop was, I think, a step further down the line from the much vaulted 'wall' one might anticipate 'hitting' during hard physical effort. It was, quite simply, the body saying "no". Nonetheless, after a couple of hours, things again looked a little brighter (I was at least awake) and, again, draped unceremoniously and rather shakily across my trusty bike, I managed another 40 or so miles to our destination for the night - I am nothing if not determined once I have an end in sight.

Again, lots of food and a little rest helped to shore up my failing legs and we eventually arrived, some three of four days later, at John O'Groats without too much further incident (for those yet to visit this geographic outlier, I must admit to being singularly underwhelmed by this quite literal 'end of the road').

It is, ironically, sometime after the end of the ride that the story I intend to tell really starts, for not long after the ride was completed I found myself experiencing physical problems that could no longer be ignored and I have, in the intervening years been diagnosed with Systemic Sclerosis (Scleroderma) and Addison's Disease, both potentially life-limiting auto-immune conditions, either of which would fully explain the difficulties I experienced on the End to End ride. Given the potential seriousness of either condition, I am surprised I did not experience more difficulty and feel lucky to have been able to complete the End to End, and many other, significant physical challenges in years past.

I guess the critical point of my meanderings is that, had I known then what I know now about the dangers of over exertion, particularly with Addison's disease, I feel certain I would not have been sufficiently courageous to undertake the End to End ride. I would have been fearful of losing control of a body that is (now at least) demonstrably untrustworthy and increasingly unable to respond well to any physical challenge presented to it. But… I did *not* know, so ignorance was, if not bliss, then at least a factor which mitigated towards a 'yes' rather than an automatic 'no' when it came to taking on a challenge that might, at first sight, have seemed impossible.

Nowadays, however, I can make no claim to ignorance of either condition and that 'no' is pretty much automatic, as I am very cognisant of the problems that will inevitably ensue if I am to say yes to any sort of hard physical challenge. This will be a familiar scenario to anyone living with a long-term condition; often the impact of saying yes is simply too great and one is impelled to live a life of physical limitation and the frustrations (at the very least) that this inevitably generates. There will be those who claim that these limitations are self-imposed, whatever the nature of physical illness, but I would counter that an assessment of what is, and what is not, possible can only be reliably

183

made by the individual who experiences that condition day in and day out.

What I can guarantee for myself now is that I won't be doing another end-to-end ride, another coast-to-coast walk or another mountain marathon (all of which I have successfully completed in the past), but what writing this short piece (and reading other people's contributions) has enabled me to do is to look forward, rather than back, with a view to setting realistic goals and working towards them in small, incremental, steps. Any resulting achievements will be tiny in comparison to most, if not all, of the other contributors here, but 'challenge' is understood, experienced and undertaken profoundly differently by everyone and one should certainly not measure one's own achievements by other people's standards – therein only lies an inevitable sense of inadequacy and failure.

Most importantly, I'm grateful for the opportunity to commit these reflections to paper, as what this process has generated, for me at least, is a renewed determination to challenge myself within the boundaries that illness inevitably imposes. I hope that, whatever your own abilities and/or limitations, you might consider doing the same, because the satisfactions to be gained from achieving even the most mundane or seemingly inconsequential goal are immeasurable.

First up, then, I've paid my money and signed up for a short sportive ride of only 25 miles (which, as I write this in early January 2018, might as well be 250) and, in the spirit of Team Avago, I'll certainly let you know how it goes.

Gareth

My sister, I'm so proud of you and I'm grateful to you for helping me get this book finished. My friends are special to me and I'm hoping to have the chance to give more of them a chance to write their stories with a view to inspiring others to 'avago!

This book is the result of my sister saying the same to me as I'm saying to you, 'What's stopping you, do it!'

It's a cliché I know, but I'm slamming it in now. Why assume something is going to fail until you've tried it? Why not enjoy doing it, the thing you've always dreamt of, just enjoy it and then see what happens, listen to those words of Goethe, really ingest them and have a think and, if you need a little more help, read on.

My friend Jackie might just tip you over the edge into a whole new chapter in your life.

Jackie Gavin - Ironman Diary of a Menopausal Woman

Friday 25th July 2014 after my morning spin class

Me to Gareth who'd just finished Ironman "I could never do that"

G, he throws me a quizzical look

Me 'Don't you be planting seeds!'

G '19th July 2015, just saying'

A couple of texts followed, so to humour G I told him the seed was planted so let's see. I would break it to him later that it's thanks, but no thanks. I could not possibly complete Ironman.

V1ntage gym is run by Gareth, who, having, said he'd never do a 3rd Ironman, decided to enter a team of 10 including himself and G persisted, saying I would be a good asset to the team so, flattered that I was, I seriously (and quietly) thought about taking on such a massive challenge, secretly looking on the internet for reasons to do it or rather not to do it.

It's my big 50 next year, I thought to myself, but sadly, yet more importantly to me, my beautiful daughter would have been 18. If I was gonna do it, she would be my inspiration.

Okay, so I am ok on a bike but swimming and running? For those distances? No chance at the moment and serious training would be required. And I mean serious. Next thing, how to tell hubby? He would think I was nuts, but knowing me as he does, he would eventually come around and be very supportive of me, but we'll park that for now.

Tuesday 29th July - The 2015 Ironman team is unveiled, without me at my request, as I need to see how I fare at running before making my decision. In 2010 I couldn't run a minute on a treadmill without stopping so, to run a marathon?

Wednesday 30th July - I bite the bullet and go out jogging to see how I get on. Why am I so nervous? Fear of failing is why. Anyway, I jogged to my mums. Granted, it was only 2.6 miles but I felt good, didn't stop and could have easily carried on. So, decision made. I have a foundation, albeit a very weak one, but I've got 11 months to improve and a good support network around me to advise and guide me through. I message G to say I'm in (now got to work up courage to tell my husband). Despite signing up, I still feel sick, but realise I'm over analysing things and need to try to relax. I printed off a training plan to use as a guide, proposing to start it next week and rang up our local sports centre for an induction on 7th Aug for swim and gym.

Saturday 2nd August - went out on my bike, taking in the infamous Sheephouse Lane, one of the hills on the Ironman route. The beauty of this Ironman is that the route is literally on my doorstep, so it would be criminal not to take advantage of it. I set off and have nothing, absolutely nothing, in my legs and my pace was shocking. 20 miles at 8.91 mph! I was so deflated I messaged G to discuss my disappointment. Granted I wasn't on a road bike, but it was still awful. I think my time of the month is approaching and that's where this title came to me – nearly 50 and menopausal, this should be fun!

Gareth told me not to worry and we arranged to go out the following Saturday together. Now, this is where I struggle. I feel so intimidated by his achievements and his biking skills, that I feel completely inferior. He tells me to feel the fear but do it anyway. He's right. What's to lose? I'm going to embrace this next year and think of myself as my own personal guinea pig.

Let's see how much I can achieve in just one year.

Monday 4th August - I take my road bike, purchased ages ago and only used twice due to lack of confidence, into my local shop to get it checked over ready for Saturday. I also email two work colleagues, both members of Bolton tri-club and they are both so supportive, encouraging me to join as their training would be very beneficial. Lastly for today, and most important, I work up courage and tell Ste my husband, my decision to compete in Ironman. Just one, only one "you're stupid you" and a roll of the eyes, but I don't have to peel him off the ceiling as anticipated.

So, this is it. Let the training begin!

Tuesday 5th August - I email a friend who's really into running telling her of my secret plans. Turns out she has a secret plan to do Ironman 2015, but is keeping quiet at the moment to improve her swimming and cycling. She doesn't feel the need to join a tri-club and gives me loads of great tips, including details of nearby open water swims. More food for thought!

Wednesday 6th August - I'm undertaking Ironman 2015 in aid of my beautiful daughter Mollie who would be 18 next year. Mollie passed away, aged 6 years old from leukaemia 11 years ago today. To mark this day, I am going on my first 'endurance' training run. The weather holds out and I make it round non-stop, taking in a couple of inclines, so very encouraged.

Thursday 7th August - joined my local gym on a gym and swim membership so I can use their pool and the treadmill when the weather's really bad.

Friday 8th August - first interval run before work. It was only 30 minutes and I managed it but was slower than on my endurance run! Oh well, another marker laid down to improve on. I picked my road bike up from the cycle shop ahead of tomorrow's ride.

Saturday 9th August - up at 5.30am to meet guys at 6.30am, gulp! Met up and cycled some of the Ironman loop – how fantastic to have this route on my doorstep. Took in Sheephouse Lane and cycled over to Adlington and Chorley and was encouraged by my ride. I felt I could have gone faster (only a little), but focused on building up my confidence. I know I held the guys back, but they were very kind and encouraging. Cycled approx. 40 miles in 3.5 hours, which I realise is far too slow!

Monday 11th August - my little boy Luie was born this day in 2008 and lost aged just 3 hours, so I decided to go for a run in the fresh air to clear my head. 5.27 miles in 1 hour 1 min non-stop, so, encouraged.

Tuesday 12th August - 1st swim. What a disaster! How exhausting is swimming? 2.4 miles seems way out of reach on today's performance. No technique (which improved slightly after watching a girl doing it properly).

Definitely need to go to Swimfit lessons as soon as possible. Weak!!

Wed 13th August - my cycling shoes and cleats arrived! Really not relishing going out on them, but going to wear them to spin to gain confidence in clipping and unclipping before I attempt using them on the roads.

Saturday 16th August - my first 5k Parkrun. Lots of club runners there but, as it's a timed run every Saturday, I'm going to use it to benchmark my improvement (hopefully there will be improvements). Quite a hilly route and got around in 34 mins 13 seconds. Position 201 out of 230 runners. Not great, but something to work on.

Sunday 17th August - bike ride from V1ntage studio – a couple of really rough hills and very, very windy. Need to do these hills again and again.

Wednesday 20th August - went to my first Swimfit class. Swimming element not looking great, as yet another disaster. The usual instructor was on holiday (thanks for telling me when I signed in). Hung around eavesdropping for tips she gave to other swimmers so picked up two tips. 1 how to breathe underwater (say 'bubble, bubble bubble' 3 times under water) and that my head was too low in the water. Trying to be positive in that I did learn something, but a bit disappointed in that session. She's away next week, so not coming back to that class. Will try another swim centre next Tuesday as the guy there has been recommended.

Saturday 23rd August - 2nd Parkrun – 30 seconds slower, what?! Took my road bike into the bike shop to see if it can be tweaked and upgraded and the guy there pretty much condemned it – he was very diplomatic though! He recommended 2 Raleigh bikes which would greatly improve my performance. 1 was £750 and the other £1k. Hmmm, how to break that to hubby? Left a Raleigh brochure on the dinner table for him to see as an ice breaker.

Sticking to my schedule at the moment, but it's ramping up slowly each week.

Tuesday 26th August - Swimfit instructor guy is on holiday this week! Will I ever get any help with my swimming?

Thursday 28th August - Open Water familiarization session. This is at Pennington Flash near Leigh, where the actual Ironman swim is held. Again, I am so thankful that all this is local to me. Slightly apprehensive, but getting in with my wetsuit on was ok. I didn't feel anxious about not being able to put my feet down or not being able to see the bottom, as the wetsuit kept me quite buoyant so could easily rest to catch my breath (and thoughts). Tried front crawl but mainly did breast stroke. Really enjoyed the session and as the centre is open to the public I can come along whenever I want to practice (there's a swim on New Year's Day, but might give that one a miss!). G pointed out the distance of the route and it was very daunting – it seems like such a long way. A guy at the centre said that out of the 2000 ironmen starters this year, 6 did not make the swim cut off time. I pray I make it next year!

Sunday 31st August - Manchester 100 cycle ride. I did this event last year with a friend, cycling the 100km route which is about 60 miles. I encouraged my friend to join me on the 100-mile route this year as a) we've never cycled 100 miles in 1 day and b) I wanted to see how that number of miles felt on a road bike as I previously cycled it on my mountain bike. It went well. I felt strong in my legs and core but had a terrible ache at the top of my spine and after the ride my knees were sore. I'm optimistic that with a better bike and cleats and more hill training the Ironman ride should be ok.

Monday 1st September - Monday Run Night. After yesterday my knees are still sore and I am so not in the mood for this, but meeting a friend at 6.15pm. Moaned whilst getting changed and then got a text from my friend, who was stuck at train station. Hmmm, what to do? Well, I figured that sitting on my arse is not going to get me over the finish line next July, so off I toddle. Result! 5.5 miles in 57 minutes – really pleased with myself. Another friend said to take quick baby steps so put that into action half way round and got a personal best on a section of the route (as recorded on Strava - using Strava as Mapmyride does not like my phone). Recording each ride / jog is great as it shows improvements which is very encouraging.

Tuesday 2nd October - not written in a while. Had 10 nights in Egypt 8-19th Sept and decided to do nothing whilst there. Partly guilt tripped into it by hubby and friends who don't exercise, and I was also feeling tired. Bad mistake!! Got back home Sat 20th Sept and had signed up for the Bolton Bash the next day, a 35-mile circular bike ride. The ride took in some horrendously tough hills and I really, really, struggled. I wasn't helped by my bike which failed miserably on them and helped confirm my decision to make getting a new bike a priority. Whilst I did complete it, the ride left me completely demoralized and deflated. Had I not signed up for ironman, things would have been fine, but I have, so the outcome was not encouraging! Anyway, got back on with the training but no cycling, the bike has been demoted to the turbo trainer so need to start using last year's Christmas pressie (used about 4 times this year!)

G has promoted a 10 class 10 day for 28th September, run 10 miles, do a 45-minute spin class then run home 10 miles. I am nowhere near that now so me and a friend decided on a 5.5 mile, class, 5.5 mile home. I managed it non-stop, but struggled the last part. Nonetheless, I was encouraged. May try 10 class 5 next time?

Looking at bikes is really confusing, as there are so many out there with very differing reviews. The Boardman Carbon was touted, but Halfords don't let you try them and there's no way I'm parting with £1k without a trial. Need to definitely go and sort this weekend to get back out on the road. I'm going hill walking next Saturday, so mixing up the training nicely. I was warned that people start out too eager in their training for Ironman and burn out, but feel I've got a nice balance at the moment and plan to ramp up after my holiday to Goa in January (shorts and trainers coming with me on that trip!). I went swimming on Tuesday, encouraged by hubby, as I really didn't want to go for fear of failure. I was tasked with swimming half a mile in 30 mins, as, if I do that, I can work on endurance and would complete swim within the allotted 2 hours 20 mins. I managed 800 metres in 27 minutes doing breast stroke so was chuffed with that. Not chuffed with technique, but practice will help. Oh, and ordered and received Don Fink's book about ironman, so will read that to hopefully gain some top tips and advice.

Thursday 9th October - suffering badly with a heavy head cold which has really taken it out of me and my vocal chords much to Ste's delight. Left me not feeling up to doing anything, so had a couple of days off. However, ironman countdown does not stop due to me not feeling 100%, so bit the bullet and went to lunch spin Tuesday, which was very hard. Sweated buckets and found it tough, but really pleased that I made the effort. Made the effort yesterday to go on my turbo trainer at home as I may as well make use of it. Set my turbo up and watch The Chase on TV and did 30 mins and another 30 mins this morning before work (along with Day 6 of the 30 day plank challenge – I will strengthen up this core of mine!).

A friend of mine won a 6 month gym membership at the Holiday Inn Bolton and kindly gave it to me to help with my training. Not sure how big their pool is but will take advantage and, it's open from 6.30am – 10pm so can go before and after work easily. Will utilise the weights in the gym to strengthen my upper arms and legs. Feeling positive about the challenge ahead – just need this cold to push off!

Friday 17th October - feeling something like today, which is great after 2 weeks of feeling lethargic and off. Not felt like doing much, but managed the basic studio classes to stop myself feeling completely pathetic and inadequate. I met a lady for a coffee yesterday who completed Ironman this year, which was so not a good move. She is a member of a running club and very fit with a structured Ironman training plan. The meeting left me feeling even more panicky, so asked G this morning if I can complete Ironman without having to be as focused as that lady, as I just want to complete it. He reminded me to focus on15/50/35 (% in each element), which I will do as I want to enjoy the journey, including the training without it feeling like an army drill. Promised G I would look to buy a bike a week tomorrow (off on a boozy barge trip for my nephew's 21st (booze will have to be dropped soon also).

Sunday 2nd November - me and Rhauri, my running buddy, ran 9.6 miles to gym, did a spin class, then ran 9.4 miles home (dead on my feet by the time I got home, but did it). We ran 1 of the marathon loops which wasn't bad (6 miles) and it has just one small incline so that was also pleasing. Been out running regularly having agreed to swim 2 x per week, run 50 miles per month and cycle 100 miles per month – doable at the moment.

Just gotta crack this swimming!

Friday 14th November - not written in a while, but training going well. Swimming, though, that's not going well, but will persevere with breast stroke. Thinking of investing in 1-1 swim coaching to improve my technique. I cycled a loop of the Ironman route on Sunday and didn't sleep well the night before and was really nervous getting picked up. I commented that it would either motivate or demotivate me. I actually enjoyed it, finding that it was quite flat in some parts which would mean I would be able to bat along to claw some time back on

the day. Obviously, Sheephouse was a killer, but
Hunters Hill, the other beast climb, was not as bad as I
imagined. I have to remember that I only did one loop
(47.5 miles), so would need to do that again and cycle
additional miles before running a marathon! We cycled
it in 3 hrs 5, so was pleased with that as a first pass. My
bike was awesome now I have become used to the
gears. Oh yes, forgot to mention I plumped for the
Decathlon Mach 700 as I got a really good price and
read some good reviews – so far so good. I've been
advised to add an 11:32 cassette on the back to make
hills a little easier, so will invest in that next year.
Running going good too. Onward…

Doing my first brick session on Sunday - a cycle ride
followed by a (hopefully) 10 miles run. If I run that non-
stop, it will be the farthest I've managed – we'll see.
Brick session? You may well ask - just a fancy name for
a back to back session of either two or three of the Tri
disciplines.

2015 - long-time no speak! New Year – not so much a
new me? Reading the last sentence. I did my brick
session, but just under a 10 mile run. Legs were a little
slow to get going after cycling but did ok. Need to do a
run after a bike ride where possible, as told that's good
training.

I got through Xmas ok (always a painfully emotional time
for me and I seem to 'go into myself', but I survived).
Then went to Goa 6-20th Jan with friends to celebrate his
60th birthday. I said I would go running twice a week
whilst away as I do at home and managed that plus an
additional run. No swimming done as pool was too small
and the Arabian Sea's current was too dangerous.

196

Came back raring to go though and straight back into swimming on 22nd and a spin class Fri 23rd.

Week ending 31st January 2015 - did well this week, but was a frustratingly mixed week. Sunday started off with a 2 hours studio spin session as weather too bad for outdoor cycling. Monday went swimming early, but casual swimmers and old ladies chatting meant I was lane hopping (memo to self not to go too early on Mondays again). Tuesday went running on treadmill and managed 30 mins non-stop at 8-8.5kmph so really pleased with that. Thurs went swimming and did an hour non-stop (64 lengths) in 50 minutes so felt uplifted (I was thinking of going to another swim class but have decided to go it alone as completely intimidated and frightened. Met G after work for a chat, he advised I should focus more on cycling, so swapped my Friday treadmill run for a 45 min spin class. Saturday was a 4 hour hill spin session with HRM and G wanted us to emulate 4 solid hours on the bike, so food and drinks on board / to hand and no getting off unless necessary.

I set off great, but really lost it the last 40 minutes, being unable to meet the effort levels he demanded of us and with 15 mins to go thought I was going to throw up! I had taken 2 spare bottles of water with electrolytes in which I'd not used before and I ate frequently (as you're advised), but think I had taken on too much, plus, I feel like a period is coming which is wiping me out (being menopausal I can't plan them these days). I got off feeling a big loss of confidence – what if a period comes on Ironman day? Anyway, gotta get over it and move forward.

Went to our friends for a get together and our last drinkipoos before we all go 'dry' for February. Looking forward to Feb and gonna use it to build on things.

Monday 2nd February - Well, should have gone running this morning but have no energy or motivation. Must try harder!

Monday 9th February - took part in a mini triathlon from Vintage to get a feel for transition. It consisted of 400m swim, 23 mile ride and a 5k run. My swim time was 12 min 30 seconds and then out and off on bike. It was freezing! Foggy and freezing, but battled around the course in 2 hours 08, average speed 11 miles per hour (not fast enough as need to be at least 14 miles on the day). However, I wasn't too daunted and never felt like giving in, so was heartened by that. Straight off the bike onto the run, which was uphill for 1.5 miles. I think I may have been able to crawl faster initially but speeded up after a while. Completed 3.3 miles in 41 mins. I thought the guys would have been done and home before I started my run but was so pleased so see one of the gang romping home as I set off so not bad for an owd 'un! And, not aching today so, again, good result.

Friday 13th February - What a great week! After an horrendous start Monday at the pool where I had a mini meltdown, the week finished on a high. I went swimming Monday again using breaststroke and was so frustrated at my speed (my colleagues leisurely passing me whilst I was busting a gut!) Anyway, my friend Michelle entered the pool and said to invest in a nose-clip as it helped her tremendously (going from a non-swimmer last July to confidently swimming front crawl).

Bought said nose-clip at lunch with a view to trying it out at the Holiday Inn spa pool to get a feel for it, it went ok. I did 35 mins on the treadmill before my swim which, again, went well. I'm not sure whether the machine is set up in KM or miles so don't want to brag just yet but pleased with my speed and endurance. Went swimming Thursday and after the nose clip popping off and me chasing it under water as it scurried around like a little crab, it worked well. I managed single laps of crawl without panicking which was encouraging. 1 lap down, just another 159 to go! Will practice lots on my crawl (in the secrecy of the Holiday Inn to work on my breathing and bilateral technique) before trying it out in the big pool (will watch videos on YouTube for top tips). I feel I'm ramping my training up nicely and am enjoying it without feeling overwhelmed, which is exactly what I want.

Out tomorrow cycling with G and Dave Evans and then out Sunday morning Kelly. G emphasized to us all just how long we're in the saddle on Ironman day and therefore we need speed and endurance for that section – as I said, not fast enough at the moment so defo need to work on speed, particularly on the flat and downhill. Contemplating biting the bullet this Sunday and putting my cleat pedals on after our bike lesson in tyre changing – not looking forward to it, but know it's got to be done. Also, still dry and sleeping great.

Tuesday 24th February - not such a good week last week. Went on a hilly bike ride with Kelly which was only 1.5 hours long. Did great on hills but just can't get speed up on the flat, plus my saddle is leaving me very swollen, not just sore, swollen (too much information I know!). Invest in a cut out saddle to see if that helps. Went to maintenance lesson and couldn't get my tyre off, so what happens if I get a puncture on the day? Just rolling with it and keep going, doing various classes to keep the variety and overall strengthening going. Swimming again was a disaster, so signed up for Improver lessons starting tomorrow night – let's see how they go and if they help! I did have a brilliant treadmill session, running for 44:15 mins, so was really pleased with that and enjoyed run club on Saturday but, as G keeps saying, it's all about the bike.

The weather is sooo cold and foul though there's not much chance to get out on it, so doing lots of spin classes instead. G's gonna fit me a cadence computer on my bike to see if that helps me with my speed, so having that fitted tomorrow. Keeping the faith at the moment in the hope it all comes good. Got a really painful right shoulder, so got to be careful. I had a sports massage last Wednesday which was horrendous, the lactic build up in my shoulders was so painful. A guy posted on Ironman Journey Facebook page to not get hung up on the science of stuff and just enjoy training, which I thought was great advice – keep training and putting it in – easy!

Friday 13th March - had a MASSIVE Ironman wobble recently on Monday 2nd March. I went out on the bike, on my own, the weather was foul, but I'd set my mind on going out on my cleats for the 1st time so didn't want to sway from that. It was shocking. I didn't enjoy it, my pace was too slow, and I was so saddle-sore again, despite my new saddle. I went swimming the following day and my meltdown happened in the pool. I just wondered what the hell I was doing this for. I want to enjoy the journey, but it wasn't happening.

Luckily for me, my pal Michelle, came to the pool and calmed me down…again! I got out early and, after work, had a chat with Ste and decided to carry on, so ordered my wetsuit. I am totally not underestimating the challenge ahead and feel very afraid.

Sunday 8th March the Vintage crew all did a mini tri: half mile swim, 1 loop of the Ironman route, finishing with a 10k run. I was so nervous the previous night and Sunday morning but set off. The swimming went ok. G had kindly offered to cycle the route with me, despite the fact that this would slow him down. Within half a mile my chain came off and got totally wedged. Luckily, G got it loose and off we went. I struggled to keep up and again, wobble time. I thought again about quitting as the weather again wasn't kind to us (please brighten and warm up!) but, G persevered with me, giving me some good tips and, part way round, I had a lightbulb moment. I decided that I'd paid my entry, bought the bike, bought the wetsuit, so let's just train as hard as possible and turn up on the day.

After that, what will be will be. I got around the route (54 miles) in 5 hours which is too slow, but G seemed happy with that. Getting off the bike though and then running 10k was very painful, but it was a case of foot up, foot down and I did that in ninety minutes.

Home for a hot bath, hot chocolate and Soreen – lovely!

So, that's where I'm at today, back to enjoying the variety of exercise and embracing Ironman. I need to get stronger quads and leg strength, so working on overall fitness. I'm implementing my new pedal action in spin classes, resulting in aching calves, got aching butt from Tabata class, and aching quads and thighs from BLT class. My body shape is changing dramatically, but I am eating for England (I lost 4lbs doing the mini tri!). Got a 2 hour spin session tomorrow – bring it on. Come the lighter nights, I plan to get out every night if possible to cycle some hills round and about my home.

Also, did my 3rd swim lesson on Wednesday and my lovely instructor, Scott, is optimistic I can crack the crawl and do a combination of that and breast stroke on the day. Paid for 10 more lessons, so will be interested to see how I swim after that. Open water starts next month too, so hopefully that will give me some more confidence. As G says though, it really is all about the bike, so need to work really hard on that!

Got great support from family and friends which really helps. Ordered my sweat band for the run, so need to get that embroidered – Team Gav all the way!

Tuesday 14th April - long-time no speak and such a lot has happened. Positivity has not waivered and I am really enjoying this journey. I have a very varied programme with lots of core conditioning and boxing classes as well as cycling and swim classes (not much running though!). G keeps on that it's all about the bike, so been doing a lot of hill training round and about my home and feel I'm getting stronger. Did the Ironman loop again, but got massively lost which resulted in 7.5 hrs in saddle, which we survived (me and Rhian). So, we know we can do the time, just need to match that with the distance. Completed Decathlon's Duathlon Sunday 12th

April (6k run-28k bike-6k run) in 2 hours 50 mins and felt I fared ok.

It gave me good experience of transition and I came in 10 mins behind Rhian, so was pleased as she's a little powerhouse. So, just more of the same really for the next 13 weeks, but with a lot more long bike rides in with a run straight afterwards. Going open water swimming this Saturday for the first time since deciding to do Ironman and I'm seriously hoping that the buoyancy of my wetsuit allows me to swim crawl effectively. Always got breast stroke to fall back on in the worst-case scenario!

It's my 50th on the 25th April, so family putting something on, then after that, the alcohol will be pretty much zeroed out until July 19th, Ironman day. Lost lots of weight with all the training, resulting in me being able to get in a size 10 dress- who'd have thought it (current weight is 9 stone 7lbs which means I've lost exactly 4 stone since my journey began in 2010).

I have the Horwich Tri on 3rd May and cycling the C2C with some friends over 3 days in May. Planning on getting out on the hills for 1-2 hours a few nights after work now the weather and nights are lighter and brighter. Feeling optimistic – let's pray that continues.

Friday 9th May - Having a rest day today as very weary body and it's that time of the month again. I say that time of the month, but being menopausal, I never know what's happening! Anyway, I completed my first Triathlon (Horwich tri) last Sunday. My time was 3 hrs 30 mins and felt good re swim, run and transition, but bike speed still too slow and the weather hasn't helped.

As it's so cold and windy it's not been easy getting out on the bike, so lots of spin and strengthening classes to compensate.

I've no bike now for a week, as it's in the shop for an 11:32 cassette ahead of next week's Coast to Coast bike ride. I'm going to use next weekend's ride as a training event and hopefully I will gain some speed and confidence (else I'm in trouble).

I went Open Water swimming on my 50th, completing 1.15 miles in 53 minutes, so pleased with that as a starting point. The quicker the swim, the more time on the bike! I also went last Wed morning, but it was so choppy I was glad to get out (same distance and time). Going again tomorrow morning and may attempt 3 loops (4 being the 2.4 mile ironman distance). I really enjoy OW swimming much more than pool and am not planning to go to the pool other than the remaining 3 swim classes as it is so boring.

My birthday went ok with not too much alcohol consumed, but, reading people's posts on the internet, Ironman wannabees do drink, just in moderation (weird word that, moderation ha ha!). Ordered a bespoke tri-suit along with my studio eventers – just need to break it to hubby that that's another £100. Ordered a 2 piece to allow for quick toilet breaks etc.

Feeling confident, although I feel that I should be doing something every day. After next weekend's ride I really need to up my cycling and do some mini brick run sessions after – just need this weather to improve!

Tuesday 26th May - this journey is certainly full of ups and downs. Had a cracking 3 days cycling C2C. Kept up with Rick and managed some brutal hills. Really thought I was going to get blown off my bike on the exposed, bleak, open North Pennine Moors, I was seriously scared! My pace is still not up to speed, but felt I was doing ok and picked up some good tips. That seemed a long way away as a ride Sunday morning left me very frustrated. 44.5 miles in 3 hrs 30 so average speed only 12.7 mph. Took some solace knowing, again, I took on some tough local climbs and was rewarded with some improved splits on the flat (used my drops to speed along) but still frustrated.

Went out again yesterday and took on Scout Road, Edge Lane, Foxholes (hate that hill) and Sheephouse. Again, felt some improvement on the hills and whizzed down hills on my drops but 18.8 miles with average speed still only 12.9mph. My OW swim last Thursday went ok – managed 1.5 miles in 1 hour 1 minute, so if I can maintain that I would complete the swim section in 1 hr 40. At this point I need to reduce further as that would give me more time on the bike – I think I need a motorized fin!

I'm booked on an 82 mile Sportive this Sunday so, again, a good indicator of where I'm at (or a bad one!). The route takes in some of the Ironman loop, so let's see how that goes. I figure at this stage, just keep training and what will be will be as, 8 weeks yesterday, I finally get my life back

My mum is desperate for this to be over!

Monday 5th June

Did my sportive and it was hard. Drove 25 miles to Ormskirk and ended up cycling to within a mile of my home, over to Darwen and back to Ormskirk! There were some tough hills and the weather wasn't kind, so a tough day overall, but I did it in 6 hours 52 minutes and never had to get off to push, stopping only once to refill my water bottle. Went open water swimming last Thurs and did 2 x 1100m, beating my time the previous week by nearly 8 minutes and, on Saturday, the V1ntage Ironman team cycled 2 loops of the Ironman route (approx. 110 miles) and I survived! I worked hard and to the max in parts but, to be honest, there were bits of the course I could have pushed harder so, on the day what with the various elements of adrenalin, closed roads, crowds etc, I'm hoping that'll give me an extra push, so a good week overall.

I ate loads on the bike, emptying my top bag and devouring my mini pork pies from the back of my cycle jersey but I didn't feel too bad nutrition and energy wise (just a little sick). My main problem is neck ache and when bending my neck to relieve it, it feels like someone's prodding me with a red-hot poker – not pleasant, but we're not designed to sit and cycle for hours on end. Saddle soreness not too bad, but I had lumps in my groin from the previous week's ride and, having, suffered this before, required antibiotics to clear so I need to get some in time for the big day as it wasn't fun setting off with them.

I'm quietly optimistic that I can actually do this now, although it's still gonna be right down to the wire. The support and encouragement from friends, family and V1ntage members has been brilliant and my Ironman buddy Rhauri is a complete star.

I've been pool swimming this morning, but it is sooo boring I'm not going again other than my swim lessons. I'm actually enjoying the lessons, going from totally dreading it to feeling I can do whatever my lovely coach Scott asks of me. The lessons have been really great for me from both a technique and confidence boosting perspective and I would thoroughly recommend them. I'm going to focus on open water swimming from now though until the big day. I've got to go into work this Wednesday, it's normally my day off, but after that I'm going to go down 6.30am to replicate how conditions will be at that time of day. I've got an ironman training day this Sunday with Endurance Tri Club. This consists of a full 2.4mile swim plus a bit of experience of a mass start and 1 loop of the cycle route. More miles in the hurt locker, 5 weeks Sunday - eek!!

On the plus side (although hubby might not agree), the weight is dropping off me – it's hard to keep eating, which I'm doing all the time. Had a good cooking evening last night, so freezer filled with healthy soups and meals for the week.

Oh, I also did a bit of bike maintenance prior to Saturday's ride, I cleaned my bike, chain and pumped up my tyres. Still not practiced changing the tyres yet but may do that prior to it going in for pre-Ironman service on 20th June so if I cock it up they can sort me out!

Monday 6th July 2015 - Wow, so much has happened since I last wrote, where to start? I did the training day. Rocked up to 3 Sisters at Wigan for the swim and was so nervous. It's only small and we had to do 3 circuits in order to complete 2.4 miles. I set off and was really panicky, but soon settled down. People swam off away from me and I was then expecting to get lapped and overtaken by the next wave of swimmers. No-one did which freaked me out a bit as I wondered if I was swimming wrong? I completed 3 laps and looked at my watch and the time was 1 hour 27! What? Me? 1 hour 27? I was elated with that and the fact I managed it all non-stop and front crawl

From there, we all went for breakfast before setting off on the bike for a loop of the Ironman circuit. That also went well, and we cycled 80 miles in total. The following week was usual classes and swimming. I dropped my bike of for pre-ironman service and a 1.5 hour spin class Sunday. The week after, me and Rhauri tried to ramp our running up. We started running together soon after signing up for ironman but then did our own thing. We decided we'd finish this journey as we started with a Monday night run. I'd discussed with Rick from running club the run walk technique which he endorsed in order to complete and survive a marathon, so we put that into practice. The issue was trying to find the right ratio for us. We started out at 5 min run 1 min walk but upped it to 8 minute run, 2 min walk, and we completed 8.9 miles in 1 hour 39 (it was hilly!). As my bike was still in the shop, we went out running Thurs instead of our usual ride and we ran 10 min, walked 2 minutes and we did 11 miles in 2 hours, which was very pleasing.

Saturday 28th June - was another training day with Invictus Tri Club. That was a swim at the Delph, a 2 Ironman loop and run after. Went along and swim started at 7.30 but needed to be out and ready to cycle at 9, so only managed 1.5 miles in 47 minutes (still pleased). Set off on the bike in Group 2, the middle group, and really struggled. Just did not feel the love and my legs were weary. I was very teary too due to my daughter, Mollie's upcoming 18th birthday on Tuesday, and contemplated binning off the 2nd loop, however I gave myself a serious ticking off and buckled down. I thought I'd drop back into the 3rd group, but we couldn't even catch them up! We did catch them eventually, which made me feel a little better as I wasn't last anymore, but I was glad to get the ride done (96 miles in 8 hours which included lots of stops) we finished with a 5k run which I did in 30 minutes and was pleased with that too having just cycled (I'm easily pleased aren't I!).

The day did not do anything for my confidence as I still felt I was too slow and the bike cut off starting to freak me out. Texted my mentor G for a chat and arranged to meet on Thursday for a coffee.

Managed a run the following night with Rhauri which surprised me as I felt ok – just our usual 5.27 mile route, although he went on to run further. I would have, too, but friends were visiting us. My daughter's 18th on 30th June completely floored me more than it usually did, but I made myself get out on the bike and I did 10.5 miles on the bike with an average speed of 14.4 mph – that ride was for my girl, I didn't make my swim lesson on Wednesday as my heart wasn't in it but managed a spin class.

I met G for a coffee and he suggested I do a non-stop loop on my own to see how I fared. I immediately dismissed this, as I had done my last big bike ride before taper, however this was another seed planted! I decided that I would have a go to banish my demons on Sunday morning with no traffic about.

Saturday 4th July - I went OW at Penny Flash as they've now opened the actual swim route, so I swam 1 loop of that – it seemed a long way and it was difficult to sight. I'm going to go again this Wed to familiarize myself with it.

Sunday 5th July - got up at 5 to drive to the start of the loop. Set off at 6am and went hell for leather. It was a lovely day and virtually no traffic so no stops except for 3 traffic lights. I'd booked on to a spin class at 11 and wanted to get back for that and I did the ride in 3 hours 16 minutes, just over 14mph which, if I can maintain that speed (and that would be tough) would get me to cut off!!

Home for a quick shower and food then out to spin. I didn't think I would have much in my legs, but I felt good and strong which was very encouraging. So, all in all, a great weekend for me and demons banished for now. Sadly, learnt that Dave Evans had to go to hospital due to a blood infection, so fingers crossed he'll be ok for the 19th as he's worked so hard for this, even learning to swim from scratch especially!

Monday 6th July - all caught up now and its taper time. Going to try to eat more and sleep more to re-energize. Out for a run tonight with Rhauri and hope he's feeling a little brighter as he felt he had a bad weekend (a full swim and 60 miles on the bike…I don't think so).

Monday 13th July - another dodgy ride on the rollercoaster that is ironman. Did a hilly run last Monday which went well, Bounce class Tues and spin and swim

Wed – all great then Thursday came. Did turbulence class which was good but a short ride. Thursday night completely winded me – I had absolutely nothing in my legs which scared the hell out of me. Sacked the ride off after 7.5 miles and did a quick 1.25 mile run but I was scared.

Decided to cancel Friday morning spin and no classes next week to try to recover. G not happy I cancelled class, but obviously understood why.

Saturday 11th July - did 2 loops of OW swim course in 1:36 so happy with that, but swimming is very lonely and it's hard to keep your mind occupied. Met up with the team for chat about the logistics of registering and G imparted knowledge about the process and transition – was nice to chill and chat with them all without any lycra on. Decided to go and register and attend the briefing together and then rack bikes up on Saturday.

This is now very real.

Monday 13th July - did a 5k Muddy maniac course yesterday with my sis and bud which was good, light-hearted fun and just what I needed. Planned an easy ride and run with Rhauri later and am dreading how I'll feel when I get on my bike – good I hope?

Thursday 16th July - Last day at work and took in some Ironman cupcakes as a thank you to my colleagues who have supported me during my training, for listening to me fears, building me up and generously donating to my charity, The Compassionate Friends. When I lost Mollie and Lucy in 2003 I could barely get out of bed so to have come through all that and now be here, ready to tackle Ironman UK after months and months and hours and hours of training is something I could never have imagined.

Where I have found the mental strength and determination from is beyond me, but I am so thankful for my stoicism in surviving the worst tragedy that could befall a parent and doing so in such a positive way.

Friday 17th July - Met with the team for breakfast and registration. It was a positive experience in the main, chatting informally and excitedly. Sadly, one negative memory will stick with me whilst I was sharing my fears of not being fast enough on the bike leg of the race and missing the cut off (something that's concerned me throughout my training). As part of this team I have done my best to boost people's confidence when they were feeling scared or low (despite my own insecurities) and on this occasion, so near to race day, the response back to me was "my fear is I'll go too fast". Not helpful or constructive but, at the end of the day, I realise that it's me, myself and I and not anyone else's responsibility to help boost my own ego.

We all walk over the Macron to register and I am super excited. I get my race bag containing all I need for the big day and a team photo is taken. There is merchandise on sale, but I refrain from buying anything as I'm not taking it for granted that I will complete this as anything could go wrong on the day and I've never been a presumptuous person.

When home, I lay everything out in Mollie's room and meticulously fill my various bags with my equipment and food etc. I transfer my Ironman race number on my arm and look quite the part!

Saturday 18th July - Time to take my bike up to Pennington Flash to rack it up for tomorrow. I follow Rhauri up and we park up on the busy field. So many competitors busy making last minute adjustments to their bikes ahead of tomorrow. We rack ours up and bump into G, just arriving. He shows up the transition tent and talks about the process. This year is the first year the swim is self-seeded, so we look at where we are going to place ourselves. I figure 1 hour, 45 minutes for me but secretly hoping for a slightly better time (the faster the swim, the more time on the bike!).

Being lucky enough to live in Bolton has enabled us to practise and practise swimming the actual course but people come from all over the world to take part in this event, so they are using today as a familiarisation of the course. We watch as they swim in very choppy waters, I'm hoping the water will be calmer tomorrow.

I head home for a chill day but just pottered around as I was too pent up to sit and watch a boxset or something as G had suggested. An early start tomorrow as me and Rhauri are booked on the bus from the Macron at 4am to take us up to the Flash. An early start for Ste too as he's kindly volunteered to drive us up there, but the difference is he gets to go home and back to bed whilst I embark on the biggest physical challenge of my life!

Sunday 19th July - RACE DAY!

Hardly slept through excitement and apprehension and

was awake from 2.30am. Checked in on Facebook and we're all sent so many messages of support. I felt really great and was looking forward to today.

We arrive at the Macron in the pitch black and board the bus. It drops us quite a way away, so we follow the trail of people over the fields until we reach the Flash and meet up with the rest of the team. This is it! There is a real feeling of excitement and the various teams and tri-teams gather together in their bespoke gear. We all look great in our V1ntage team tri suits (Ste finally forgave me for forking out so much for mine).

6am approached, so it was time to put on our wetsuits and start to get in line. Rhauri, Rhian and I self-seed at 1 hour 45, so make our way to the relevant flag.

I see Neil from work ahead of me and he wishes me luck. Neil has completed numerous Ironman races and is looking for an improved time as his ultimate goal is to race in Kona. My goal is simply to finish!

The Ironman song starts up, AC/DC's Thunderstruck and I shudder. I've been a big AC/DC fan since I was a teenager but never thought this song would go on to have such new meaning to me now.

The professionals start the race by entering the water first and we slowly make our way up. I hug Rhian and Rhauri and thank them for being great training buddies and wish them good luck. I have absolutely no fear and can't wait to get in. I put my goggles on and am just about to enter the water when I hear someone squeal out my name. I look to my right and there on the ramp is

Donna from work. I give her the biggest smile and wave which she captured on camera. It remains one of my favourite photos ever.

I jump into the water and it is so warm, almost bath like. A mad scramble ensues with arms and legs stopping me from creating a rhythm and I'm kicked in the ribs, hard! I keep going and crack on. Whilst learning to swim and swimming at the flash, spotting was not my strong point and I regularly found myself way off course, trying to spot the small buoys but, today, the buoys are huge, and I easily maintain a straight course. Whilst the swim is 2.2 miles it is actually 2 laps of a 1.1 mile loop so you get out, run over the timing mat and then enter the water for a second time. I swim easily and get out to re-enter the water but slip on the jetty and make the most ungraceful entry. Any spectators seeing me must have nudged each other and laughed.

During this second loop it starts to rain heavily but it makes no difference to me as I'm wet already. The melee of swimmers has petered out and I have lots of space around me and can see the finish point in front of me. I am really enjoying this, but am suddenly attacked by a swimmer from my left. He swims right over me and I come up spluttering wondering where the hell he is headed to as he is way off course and heading towards the boathouse! Not my problem today.

I gather myself and carry on and jump out of the water having completed the first section. I pass Donna again and ask her what time it is but didn't hear her reply as I was headed off to transition 1. I grab my bag and head off to change into my cycling gear and grab something to eat. I run for my bike and am shouted at when walking out with my race number not visible. I sort it and carry on running out, so I can mount my bike in the allocated area and off I go. I'm feeling really good at this point and cycle on in a bit of a blur following the route signs.

Whilst cycling up Regent Road I hear someone shout 'V1ntage' and look to the right of me to see G's wife, waving at me. I give her a wave back and carry on. A few miles later, I turn right into Babylon Lane which is heaving with public supporting the riders. I hear my name again, this time from Donna from the gym, who's sat watching from her front door step. Onwards towards Rivington and Sheephouse Lane for the first time. I've cycled this many times during training, having had both good and bad days.

This loop is one of the good day variety and I reach the bend where the V1ntage supporters are. As I approach I hear someone shout in surprise "it's Jackie", probably expecting me to be at the back of our team which made me feel good. My crew of family and friends were supposed to be with them at this point, but they are nowhere to be seen. I carry on towards Belmont and see them further along the road. They're waving and cheering at me as I approach them and all I do it shout at them that they're at the wrong point!

I drop down to the Black Dog for the sharp left turn up towards Belmont and cheery Donna from work, is there again with her lovely smile and she shouts that I'm doing fantastic. As I get to Belmont Sailing Club I feel something pop at the side of my left calf and I say out

216

loud to myself that that is not good but carry on regardless.

Belmont Road is a fabulous, long open road and cyclists are passing me in droves. I see Rhian pass me and shout out well done to her. Rhauri passes me and I shout his name, he slows down to have a quick word, but I tell him to get going. Dave Evans passes me and shouts out that he survived the swim, punching the air triumphantly. There are various rules in Ironman, one of them is no drafting and with hindsight I think I put too much energy in trying not to break any rules, to my own detriment. I'm not that clever a cyclist to even think about taking advantage of this practice and should have simply concentrated on just cycling as I feel it used up some mental energy which could have been put to better use elsewhere.

I reach Hunters Hill, the second dreaded hill on the course and the band and supporters are out. A supporter shouts "great cadence mate", unfortunately not to me, as I battle on!

Whilst the route is well supported, there are a lot of rural spots with no support and you're on your own with only you to motivate yourself. I reach Sheephouse for the second time but am really struggling this time around. As I reach the top, Ste runs down a little to run back up alongside me. I tell him I'm struggling, and he points to the 3 mini photos of Mollie, Lucy and Luie I taped to the post of my handlebars and shouts at me to do it for them. I want nothing more and push on, but am finding it so tough.

Once again I'm on the long, open Belmont Road, this time round quite alone as all the cyclists are now in front of me. I'm cycling as hard as I can with my head down and the next minute, I'm on the floor. What the hell? I look up to see another female cyclist apologising for having pulled out without looking back resulting in me suffering my first ever fall off my bike.

Great timing for that!!

I remount and carry on, but am slipping back and, looking at my watch start to fret I'm not going to make cut off, but carry on anyway. It's gonna be alright and I think back to last year when one of the girls made the cut off by 7 minutes and thought I'm gonna smash that record and scrape in with probably seconds to spare!

Unfortunately, at the bottom of Hunters Hill, 97 miles into the ride, at 3.35pm, a white van stops in front of me and apologetically tells me to pull over.

No, no no.

I only have 15 miles to go and, by my reckoning, would have just scraped home but stupidly I pull over, with another cyclist, Dwight, to wait for the recovery van. Three other cyclists walk back down the hill having also been stopped and we wait, and wait, and wait for 50 minutes for the recovery vehicle to arrive. We chatted whilst waiting and Dwight said this was his second attempt having failed last year and he would be trying again next year. One rider completed it last year but felt grim this year and couldn't make it. The other two riders struggled, and the poor guy was almost hypothermic waiting to be picked up so long. They said one girl cycled on refusing to stop and I subsequently learned it was the girl who knocked me off my bike and just scraped through to finish.

I wish so much I had carried on just to see if I could have made it in and, if not, how close I would have been. Also, it was never my plan to meet up with my waiting supporters via a van and I was devastated not to have cycled in triumphantly to their cheers. I always said my cycling speed was going to be tight and I would have been delighted and relieved to get through whatever the time.

Sadly, today was not a good day at the office.

December 2017 Gareth Price

Back in 2016, I'd asked Jackie to finish her Ironman story for me but she'd said it was still too painful. On that day, I began what was to be the last run of my Ironman journey, I'd begun to wonder where Jackie was back on the cycle course. I knew my the rest of our team were either on the run by that time or were going to be safe through the cycle cut off time.

I spent the entire run not know what had happened to her and it upset me for long periods of my marathon, as I was not certain she was ok.

Look, selfishly I wanted all 6 of us to get our finisher's medal, but I'd backed Jackie above all of them to finish, I knew her cycling was going to be the biggest part of the challenge and spent twelve months preaching at her about it. What was for sure though, she gave it everything, I always knew that!

As I trudged backwards and forwards, in and out of Bolton I was picking up stories that she'd been knocked off the bike but heard nothing of the broom wagon incident. The writing was on the wall, though, something had gone wrong for Jackie because nobody had seen her on the run. The run route meant you saw everyone multiple times. Ironman was playing a harsh trick on her team mates, but it was nothing compared to the brutal way that broom wagon treated Jackie.

She eventually put pen to paper for me and here are her reflections on her post-Ironman experience.

Jackie's story continued…

My friends and family were wonderfully supportive and we somehow all ended up back at my house where I took a quick shower whilst Ste ensured everyone was given a drink. If truth be told, there was a bit of an elephant in the room as people didn't quite know how to handle my disappointment, especially when Sylvia, an elderly lady from my TCF group, rang to check up on me.

Sylvia lives off Chorley New Road and was waiting to cheer me on with the plaque she'd made for me. She was worried having not seen me and tears streamed down my face as I told her I didn't make it, but she again was so lovely, telling me how marvellous I had done in undertaking this mammoth challenge.

I felt worse as she'd gone around to all her neighbours and raised over £200 for my charity. As much as I'm disappointed for myself, my greatest disappointment is that I've let down all the lovely people who'd donated their hard-earned money.

Sam, my sister, presented me with a medal and a card telling me how proud she was of me which meant the world to me. Since losing my children, my whole perspective on life has changed and I truly, truly value my friends and family who continue to be a wonderful source of support to me and Ste.

People trailed away, and I went to bed completely drained.

Monday 20th July 2015 - I'd pre-booked the day off work, hoping I would be at home with aching limbs

having completed ironman, instead I woke up still feeling
so devastated. G texted me, but I replied saying I was
unable to speak as I was so down.   My boss also
texted, and I replied to say that in the grand scheme of
my life, this loss was nothing, but it still hurt. It was the
first time I'd failed in anything I'd set out to do and I
didn't like it one bit.

January 2018 – Gareth asked me to complete the story
of my ironman journey which I've done, but I feel I need
to add where my thoughts are some 2 ½ years on. I feel
complete and utter pride in what I did. Looking back, I
cannot believe I had the motivation to put in so many
hours of training, doing sportives, getting up early every
day to undertake some sort of physical challenge, many
of which took me completely of out my comfort zone and
focussing 100% on my challenge, sacrificing time with
Ste, family and friends in order to succeed.

Many people tried to bolster my ego immediately after
the event, telling me how marvellous I had done in
signing up for Ironman and putting in the effort I did. I
didn't believe them at the time but now, where there are
always days I struggle to motivate myself, I am still
amazed and proud at what I achieved.

I didn't get bitten by the triathlon bug, to the great relief
of my family and friends, but now stay fit and healthy by
doing what I love; walking outdoors, spending time on
my spin bike and various other classes. My one regret is
that Ironman completely dented my confidence in
cycling and were I would love to be out every weekend, I
now struggle to find the motivation to mount my lovely
road bike. I spent so long cycling with my head down,
checking cadence and speed I've forgotten how to

simply enjoy my bike and being outdoors and this is something I plan to rectify in 2018.

For anyone wondering, should I? Whatever the challenge, do it, try it! Whatever the outcome, I guarantee you will absolutely love the journey!

What's left to say?

I think you'll agree, Jackie's story is a roller coaster ride of emotions and milestones. Why did I put it in the final chapter of the book, well, I think Jackie's Ironman illustrates so many of the aspects of team Avago.

Not least, I hope her Ironman story humanises and normalises what, for many people, is a very tall order, an ultra-triathlon which, in her case, resulted in her never getting to hold the finishers medal, but in fact, having something far more important. She's got the memories of that year in her life, which nobody can take away. A medal is great, but it's only a possession.

I, along with Dave, Andrew and Callum never got our Tour du Mont Blanc medals either, but we did some amazing stuff as we got ready to give it a go and, then, failure turns into success just as soon as you realise it's not just the taking part that counts, it's the giving of your best and knowing in your mind, nobody else's mind or eyes, how hard you tried!

If you push yourself hard enough, you'll win some and you'll lose some, if you win them all are you pushing yourself hard enough I ask you? If you enjoy your success and learn to cope with failure you'll be a better person for it

Go on, Avago, live it and take it to the edge!